"BOSS Series"

Radiology, Radiotherapy and Oncology

Dear Reader!

We have produced another wonderful text "BOSS Series" on the Radiology, Radiotherapy and Oncology with the help of most experienced and versatile author R.N. Prasad. The author has taken great pain in making this book. The recent trend in PGMEE/PGMAT examination can be successfully solved by reading this book. The chapters itself help you to solve problem-oriented clinical cases asked now-a-days in different PGMEE examinations of All India, AIIMS, PGI, State PGMAT, NIMHANS, BHU and many more like BPSC and UPSC etc.

Publisher

"BOSS Series"
Radiology, Radiotherapy and Oncology

R.N. Prasad
BSc (Dist), MBBS (Ran), MD (Pat) (Patho and Microbiology), DC Path (Pat), DCH (Pat)

Tutor-cum-Assistant Professor
Department of Pathology
A.N. Magadh Medical College
Gaya, Bihar (India)

Formerly Medical Officer
at Patna Medical College and Hospital
Patna, Bihar (India)

Ex-Tutor J.L.N. Medical College
Bhagalpur, Bihar (India)

PEEPEE
PUBLISHERS AND DISTRIBUTORS (P) LTD.

"BOSS Series"–Radiology, Radiotherapy and Oncology

Published by
Pawaninder P. Vij

Peepee Publishers and Distributors (P) Ltd.
Head Office: 160, Shakti Vihar, Pitam Pura
Delhi-110 034 (India)

Corporate Office: 7/31, Ansari Road, Daryaganj
Post Box-7243, New Delhi-110 002 (India)

Ph: 55195868, 9811156083

e-mail: peepee160@yahoo.co.in

e-mail: peepee160@rediffmail.com

www.peepeepub.com

First Edition: **2006**

ISBN: 81-88867-65-9

Printed at
Lordson, C-5/19, Rana Pratap Bagh, Delhi-110 007

to
the sacred memory
of
my father!

PREFACE

The present treatise under "BOSS Series" naming *"BOSS Series"—Radiology, Radiotherapy and Oncology* has come up to bridge the gap between those who are marathon runner to 100 metres. In fact it has come up also as per recently adopted MCI curricula and syllabus.

This book contains a comprehensive outline of the scientific principles and phenomenology that underpin the field of Radiology, Radiotherapy and Oncology. In each chapter, the author has attempted to highlight what are considered as the key concepts and pertinent facts.

The book is divided into 17 chapters covering the whole of the *"Radiology, Radiotherapy and Oncology"* as per recent examination trends. This treatise has been made in such a manner that students will derive the enormous quantities of factual knowledge not only in Radiology, Radiotherapy and Oncology but in relation to *Medical Sciences* on the whole.

Besides that students will find it a useful guide to go through their *"University"* as well as "*Internal assessment"* examination (Viva voce) quite comfortably fetching highest marks.

Lastly but not the least should be used by PGMAT/PGMEE service aspirants in understanding Radiology, Radiotherapy and Oncology as a whole. Even practising doctors will find this book as a good companion to deal effectively with their day-to-day more complex clinical problems.

R.N. Prasad

CONTENTS

1

Principles of Radiological Diagnostic Imaging

INTRODUCTION

- Now-a-days following modalities of diagnostic imaging are available.
  - i. Roentgen or 'X' rays.
  - ii. Ultrasound (US).
  - iii. Computed tomography (CT scan).
  - iv. Magnetic resonance imaging (MRI).
  - v. Nuclear imaging (NI).
  - vi. Radiographic contrast media (RCM).

i. Roentgen or 'X' rays

- These are electromagnetic radiation that are capable of causing "IONIZATION" in matter due to its high energy content.

> **Note:** *In HUMANS, the ionization may cause damage to DNA and cells, but it can also penetrate the body to allow non-invasive visualization of the internal anatomy.*

- X-rays can exhibit particle-like behaviour and the individual X-ray "particles" which are nothing but are discrete packets of pure energy, are called "PHOTONS".
- When an electron in an "ATOM" makes a transition from an outer orbital to an inner orbital, radiation is emitted. The emitted radiation can be visible, ultraviolet or X-ray portions of the electromagnetic spectrum.

- If an **electron beam** is accelerated toward and hits a metal target, a shower of radiation is produced by the interaction.
- In **diagnostic radiology,** X-rays are produced by a vacuum tube device called the X-ray tube. The tube contains a **tungsten** filament (cathode) and a metal target (anode), also usually made of tungsten. The filament is heated with an electric current, and a high voltage is placed between the anode and the cathode. The high voltage causes electrons in the filament to be drawn off and accelerated toward the anode. When they strike the anode, BREMSSTRAH LUNG and characteristic X-rays are produced. The "X-ray" tube is completely surrounded by **lead** on all sides, except for a small exit port. The lead absorbs most of the emitted X-rays except for the portion that escapes through the port. These X-rays are used to create the radiograph.
- The types of image receptors used in diagnostic radiology is—
  i. Storage phosphor screens.
  ii. Direct digital read out devices.
  iii. Photographic film, coupled with an intensifying phosphor screen.
- To generate high quality diagnostic radiograph, these should be—
  i. Scatter control.
  ii. Proper radiographic technique.
  iii. Technical image quality control program.
- **Fluoroscopy**
  - It is a real-time radiography.
  - Radilogists would view the light image emitted from the screens directly, as the patient was exposed.
  - Modern fluoroscopy systems use an X-ray image intensifier, which converts the X-ray energy to visible light and is coupled optically to a T.V. camera. The fluoroscopic image is viewed on a cathode ray tube video-monitor,

located either in the fluoroscopy room beside the patient or else in a remote location.

> ***Note:*** *The advantages of a modern angiography system include that small vessels can be seen using fluoroscopic equipment capable of high spatial resolution, large fields of view, and rapid digital acquisition of images.*

- **Digital subtraction angiography**
  - Images acquired after the administration of an iodinated contrast agent are subtracted from an image obtained before contrast was injected. The subtraction removes the appearance of stationary anatomy from the resulting images and synthesizes a sequence of images containing only contrast in the blood vessels. Each image in the sequence reveals a different stage in the filling of vessels with contrast.

> ***Note:*** *The technical developments that have made digital subtraction angiography possible include–small focus, high output X-ray tubes, advances in X-ray image intensifier technology, fast computers, and high-speed, large-capacity computer disk drives.*

- **The potential harmful effects of diagnostic radiology**

  i. **Stochastic effects** in which the probability of occurrence increases with radiation exposure.

  ii. **Deterministic effects** with the lowest dose threshold is early transient erythema, with a threshold dose in the 2 to 3 gray range when delivered acutely.

> ***Note:*** *The gray or Gy, is a unit of absorbed dose equal to one joule of energy absorbed per kilogram of tissue.*

- When the radiation exposure spread over-time, the threshold dose is greater than for an acute exposure, due to the ability of cells to repair non-lethal radiation damage.
- Typical doses in mGy for a following views are as follows—

a. PA view of chest- 0.15 mGy b. AP view cervical spine - 0.95 mGy c. AP view abdominal film-3.0 mGy.	Using a grid and 400 speed film, for an average patient.

- Approximately 10,000 chest X-ray or 100 CT studies or greater than 30 mts. of fluoroscopy would one need to receive before the **erythema dose threshold** is reached, if 1 Roentgen of entrance skin exposure results in a skin dose of approximately one (1) cGy.
- There is some legitimate reason to be concerned about **stochastic effects,** since they have no known dose threshold. This implies that even the smallest amount of radiation exposure may increase the probability of the induction of a stochastic effect. However, the most common stochastic effects have a fairly high spontaneous incidence, so there may be a radiation dose below which further reduction in radiation dose does not reduce the likelihood of producing the effect. Since such "negligible risk" levels have not been determined, the conservative approach is to assume that all radiation exposure to potentially harmful.
- The average annual occupational effective dose that radiologists (0.71 millisievert) and X-ray technician (0.96 m sievert).

> ***Note:*** *These exposures are much more below than the natural background exposure that is about 3.2 millisievert per annum.*

- **Radiologists and X-ray technicians** receive an average annual occupational effective dose **well below the occupational limit** of **50 millisievert/year to the whole body.**
- The health care workers who are most likely to approach the occupational limit includes **angiographers** and **cardiologists,** who perform fluoroscopically guided diagnostic and interventional procedures.
- The **main principles of radiation protection** is time, distance and shielding (lead garments and lead line partitions).

> ***Note:*** *The distance rule is particularly effective, since radiation exposure varies inversely with the square of the distances from the radiation source.*

- The standard **0.5 mm lead aprons** reduce radiation exposure by almost **95%.**
- Principles should be maintained while working with radiation or around radioactive materials to reduce exposure.
  i. Exercise proper hygiene (no drinking or eating).
  ii. Limit the X-ray field to only the anatomy of interest.
  iii. Use any dose-saving features like fast screen-film combinations, pulsed or slow-scan video fluoroscopy, or low-dose fluoroscopy whenever possible.
  iv. Use digital image receptors to reduce the number of radiographic studies that must be repeated because of under exposure or overexposure.

ii. Ultrasound (US)

- **Introduction:** US is a method of imaging that uses high frequency sound waves beyond the range of human hearing to image structures inside the body. Tissues differ in their ability to transmit sound. When a sound wave encounters a change in tissue, some of the sound is transmitted, and some is reflected to the transducer.

> **Note:** *It is the reflected sound that is converted into an image.*

- Based on the length of time it takes for the sound waves to return to the transducer, the depth of the tissue interface can be estimated.
- US waves are generated by applying an electric field to a piezoelectric crystals in the transducer, the crystals vibrates and generates sound waves. The transducer also functions as a detector, which receives the echoes reflected from within the patient.
- An US examination is performed to transmit the sound waves from the hand held transducer into the patient, a thin layer of gel is placed on the skin to serve as a coupling medium. There is no discomfort for the patient during the examination.

> **Note:** *No harmful effects of diagnostic US have been documented till todate.*

- There are several methods of US images displayed and recording. In one of the most commonly used methods, **B-mode**, the intensity of the echoes reflected to the transducer is proportional to the whitening of the film.

> **Note:** *ANECHOIC structures, which have no internal echoes, appear black.*

- **Transverse images** are oriented as if the viewer were looking upward from the patients feet.
- **Longitudinal images** are displayed with the patients head toward the left side of the image and the feet to the right.
- **Doppler US** is based on the principle that sound reflected by a moving target (e.g. **blood**) has a different frequency from the incident sound wave. This frequency shift is proportional to the valocity of the flowing blood.

> **Note:** *Dopler US, therefore, not only allows the detection of flowing blood but also enables the valocity to be quantified.*

- Colour coding the Doppler information and super imposing it on a real-time B-mode image facilitates identification of vessel and abnormal flow.
- The body structures that cannot be imaged by US includes **air containing structures** (lungs) and **bone** cannot be imaged with US.
- **Recognised advantages of US over other imaging modalities.**
  - Relatively cheaper
  - Widely available
  - Non-invasive
  - Non-radiational

  Owing to above qualities US is widely used as diagnostic tools amongst children and pregnant women.
- **Recognised disadvantages of US compared with other imaging tools.**
  - US is an operator dependent, problem-oriented modality.

  > **Note:** *It should not be used as a total body survey.*

  - US cannot image air-containing structures or bone.
  - Resolution of US image is inversely related to depth of penetration. Image quality in OBESE patient is therefore suboptimal.

iii. Computed Tomography (CT)

- **Introduction :** CT or CAT scan is a technology that utilizes X-rays to generate cross-sectional (axial) images.

> **Note:** *Any portion of the HUMAN BODY can be imaged by CT.*

- Recently introduced CT scanning can obtain an image of a transverse section of the body in one second or less.

- The X-ray beam is swept around the patient after passing through the body, the radiation strikes a series of detectors that either move with the X-ray tube or are stationary. Relatively advanced MATHEMATICAL techniques like FOURIER transformations and BACK-PROJECTION algorithms are used to create a two-dimensional image of the cross-sectional volume that is scanned.

> ***Note:*** *Although the technology is much more sophisticated than plain film radiography, the basic principle is similar–dense structures in the body block the transmission of X-rays.*

- **PIXEL Vs. VOXEL**
  Each point on a CAT image **(a pixel)** represents a small volume within the patient **(a voxel)**.
- **DENSE structures** like **metal** and **bone** are displayed **as white** on CAT scan. **Less dense** structures displayed as various sheds of **gray**, with the **least dense** structures that contain gas shown as **black**.
- The INVENTER of CAT scan is **Sir Geoffrey Hounsfield**.
- The **Hounsfield unit (HU)** is a measure of the relative density of a structure on CAT scan.

> ***Note: Water*** *(H_2O) has an HU of* ***zero*** *(0).*

- The H.U. of following structures are as follows—
  i. Minus 40 (– 40) – fat.
  ii. Positive 80 (+ 80) – soft tissue (liver on contrast enhanced CT).
  iii. Positive 400 (+ 400) – calcium/bone.
  iv. Minus 1500 (– 1500) – Air.
  v. Positive 2000 (+ 2000) – Metal.
- What is a "window"?
  Each "pixel" on a CAT image is composed of a shade of gray corresponding to the average HU

of the "voxel" that it represents. The various shades of gray create contrast in the image. The eye can appreciate only a relatively limited number of shades of gray, while the CAT data span an HU range of several thousand. To compensate for this problem, various windows are created to view optimally different structures in the body.

> ***Note:*** *To look at the lungs, a* ***wide window*** *is used.*

- For looking at abdominal structures, a much narrower window is used so that subtle differences in density are seen. The centre of the window (the level) is also set by the CAT operator.

  As for example: A typical "ABDOMINAL WINDOW" setting would be a level of + 40 (the centre HU value) and a range or width of 400 so that the CAT demonstrates all HUs between –160 and +240 as a series of shades of gray, with all pixels about 240 HU shown in white and all pixel, below – 160 shown in black.
- The typical slice thickness is 7 to 10 mm depending on the particular CT unit. This thickness is fine for most routine imaging.

> ***Note:*** *To acquire a high quality images, a higher dose of radiation must be administered.*

- **CAT scan Vs. Plain X-ray film**

i. The body is imaged cross-sectionally with CT so that complex structures can be imaged. A plain X-ray is the two-dimensional representation of a three-dimensional structure. It is often difficult to sort out overlapping structures on plain films (e.g. in the chest), and CT effectively eliminates this problem.

ii. CT is much more sensitive to differences in density than plain films are; then it can reveal abnormalities that plain films cannot.

> ***Note:***
>
> *i. A 33 years old Sangita, a patient just had a barium enema, and the referring physician now requests a CAT scan of the abdomen and pelvis; Is this a problem?*
>
> ***Ans.*** *Yes, definitely, retained barium in colon produces much more denser artefacts on CT, obscuring the normal anatomy.*
>
> *ii. Can the CT scan obtain only time axial images (images perpendicular to the CT table on which the patient rest?*
>
> ***Ans.*** *No.*
>
> *iii. A CT scan of the abdomen is ordered for a patient who developed "HIVES" in response to I.V. ionic contrast in the past. What should be done now to obtain a CT scan?*
>
> ***Ans.*** *Non-ionic contrast should be given. It may be beneficial for the patient to receive prophylactic premedication with a series of oral doses of prednisolone (50 mg orally 13, 7 and 1 hour before the CT scan) along with 50 mg of oral diphenhydramine (benadryl) one hour before the CT scan. This reduces the contrast reactions.*

- *What is SCOUT image*?
  It is a digital radiograph obtained at the start of a CT examination. It is used to obtain the axial images.
- It is important to look at this image, which contains important information (e.g. when imaging the abdomen, the bowel gas pattern should always be examined).
- Does the CAT scan table has a weight limit?
  Yes, (Many CT table has a weight limit of 300 to 350 lbs.)
- *What is a "SPIRAL" CAT*?

  Spiral or Helical CT is a major RECENT ADVANCE in CT technology. Its use eliminates the breath holding in each scan of chest, abdomen and pelvis, which is needed in conventional CT to obtain a correct scan of that area. Besides it also eliminates the resetting of scanner each time to take an scan. The X-ray tube here rotating continuously around the patient and acquire data while the patient holds his/her breath. In this way, the entire abdominal chest or pelvic organs can be scanned without changing the position or each time holding the breath.

- **In spiral CT scanner,** images can be easily reconstructed into different planes, especially if thin sections were initially obtained. Alternatively, with work stations that are connected to the CT scanner, the CT data also can be used to create more elaborate three-dimensional images.
- **CT angiography** is a new technique that can be used to study the vasculature and can be performed fairly easily and routinely with a spiral CT scanner.

> **Note:** *Is a CAT scan the samething as a CT scan?*
> **Ans**. *Absolutely right, yes.*

iv. Magnetic Resonance Imaging (MRI) or Nuclear Magnetic Resonance (NMR)

- **Introduction:** The physical principles of nuclear magnetic resonance (NMR) are the basis for MRI.
- *How is an MRI generated*?

  For this the object (patient) is placed in superconducting magnet. A strong magnetic field is created by movement of current through a series of helical coils. An electromagnetic wave or radiofrequency pulse is created through the brief application of an AC current and this "pulse" causes the H_2 nuclei of protons in the body tissues to resonate to varying degrees, thus generating a signal or an electromagnetic wave.

> **Note** : *The generated signal is based on the properties of the tissue and the settings of the magnet.*

- This signal is detected by the receiving coil, and after complex data processing an image is displayed on the monitor.

- **TESLA** is the unit of measurement of a magnetic field strength (MKS system).
- **GAUSS** is the unit of measurement of a magnetic field for the CGS system.

> ***Note :*** *One (1) Tesla (T) is equivalent to **10,000 gauss**.*

- The most common magnete field strengths used clinically are **0.3, 0.5, 1.0,** and **1.5 Tesla**.

> ***Note :*** *Magnets of 1.0 T or more are considered high field strength and generate greater signal and usually more appealing images than lower field strength units.*

- The strength of the earth's magnetic field is about 1 (one) gauss. Therefore, most MR units generate a magnetic field strength more than 10,000 times the earth's magnetic field.
- T_1 and T_2 refers to physical properties of the tissues after exposure to a series of pulses at predetermined time intervals. Different tissues have different T_1 and T_2 properties, based on the response of their H_2 nuclei to radiofrequency pulses imposed by the magnet.
- **Signal intensity** refers to the brightness of signal generated by specific tissues. Tissues that are bright (whiter) are **hyperintense**, while darker signal tissues are **hypointense**. Tissues that are in between the two are isointense.

> ***Note:*** *These terms usually refer to the signal of a pathologic process, relative to surrounding tissues (e.g. the mass is hyperintense to the adjacent muscle).*

- The term INTENSITY is used rather than the term DENSITY, which is used when referring to CT or plain films.
- The following tissues are BRIGHT or hyper-intense on T_1-weighted images and less bright on T_2-weighted images.

As for example: Fat, blood (Met Hb in sub-acute haemorrhage), proteinaceous material, melanin and gadolinium (MR contrast agent).

- The following things appear DARK on T_2-weighted images like calcium (Ca^{++}), gas, chronic haemorrhage (haemosiderin), mature fibrous tissue.
- **Water (H_2O)** is dark on T_1-weighted images and bright on T_2-weighted images. These principles are important to remember because most pathologic processes are associated with increased water content and so are **hyper-intense on T_2-weighted images** and **hypo-intense on T_1.**

> ***Note:*** *To remember it easily, a mnemonic is used like—*
> *"World War 2nd" means "Water is white on T_2."*

- What is T_R and T_E in MRI scan?
  - T_R is the time to repeat, or the time between radiofrequency pulses; T_E is the time to echo, or the time interval between applying the pulse and listening for the signal.
  - T_R and T_E are both expressed in millisecond (ms).
  - Equipment settings that elicit images that are a combination of T_1 and T_2 properties are called balanced or proton density images.
  - Looking for the T_E and T_R numbers on the images is the more difficult approach. A relatively low T_E is about **20 ms**, and high T_E is about **80 ms**, while a low T_R is about 600 ms and a high T_R is around 3000 ms.
  - T_1-weighted images have a low T_E and low T_R, whereas both are high for T_2-weighted images.
  - Proton density images have a low T_E and high T_R.
- **MRA or magnetic resonance angiography.**
  - MRI principles are used to exploit the unique properties of flowing blood. Images are

generated in which only structures containing flowing blood are visualized, all other structures are suppressed.

- These principles can further modified so that only vessels with flow in a specific direction (arteries vs. veins) are visualized.
- MRA is useful for evaluating patients with suspected cerebrovascular disease (circle of Willis or carotid arteries), and also may be applied to the venous system for evaluating suspected deep venous thrombosis.

> ***Note:*** *Definite limitations and artifacts are associated with MRA, particularly with applications outside the CNS.*

- **Recognised advantages of MRI scan over CAT scan.**

i. No ionizing radiation.
ii. Multiplanar imaging capability (axial, coronal, sagittal and oblique).
iii. Better anatomic detail.
iv. More sensitive in detecting subtle pathologic tissue alterations.
As for example—Cerebral oedema and bone marrow infiltration.
v. Improved tissue contrast compared with CT scan.
vi. Ability to characterize specific tissue types based on signal intensity.
As for example– Fat, blood and **water,** etc.

- **Recognised advantages of CAT scan over MRI (NMR) scan**

i. CAT scan is currently less expensive than MRI so **economical**.
ii. More superior for evaluating calcified or ossified abnormalities of muskuloskeletal system.
iii. CT can demonstrate the classic lesion of Paget's disease and Myositis ossificans better than MRI.

iv. CT scan is considered the modality of choice for initial evaluation of the chest, abdomen, and pelvic organs, providing high resolution anatomic changes.

v. Current CT technology allows most studies to be completed within a few minutes, compared with 30 to 60+ minutes for MRI.

vi. **Claustrophobia** is rarely a problem with the large gantry used in CT as opposed to the 10% in MRI scan.

- Is MRI safe for pregnant women?

  Ans. Not-at-all, because MRI utilizes strong electromagnetic radiation which is definitely harmful to the foetus especially during the period of organogenesis means **1st trimester**.

- **Recognised contraindications to MRI scan.** Those patients who use magnetically susceptible devices, etc. like—
  - Some penile prostheses.
  - Metal fragments (periorbital).
  - Brain aneurysm clips or coils.
  - Cardiac pacemakers.
  - Cochlear implants.
  - Some prosthetic heart valves.
  - Bone growth or neurostimulator.
  - The two gases used to cool the superconducting magnet used in MRI is Helium (He) and Nitrogen (N_2) gases.

v. Nuclear Imaging (NI)

- **Introduction: NI** is a specialised radiologic procedure in which radiopharmaceuticals are given to the patient and with the help of **gamma camera,** the images of the particular area or organs has been taken to establish the diagnosis.

> ***Note :*** *CAT scan, MRI (NMR) provide anatomic or structural information, whereas the primary purpose of nuclear imaging is to provide functional data.*

- In recent years, colour Doppler ultrasound now provides excellent images revealing blood flow; dynamic CAT scan, especially when performed with spiral technology, and MRI, if done dynamically reveal contrast enhancement in various lesions.
- Gamma rays (γ-rays) that originate from within a patient after a radiopharmaceuticals has been administered (usually I.V.) are used to form image on a **gamma camera.** In this way, nuclear images are generated.
- Recognised radiopharmaceuticals include–
  - I_2 131.
  - Technetium–99m–diethylenetriamine penta-acetic acid (T_C–99m–ĐTPA).
  - T_C 99m.
- **SPECT (Single photon emission computed tomography)**
  - It utilizes the radionuclides of standard nuclear imaging means those that emit a single photon with each radioactive decay event.
  - The term "EMISSION" differentiates the technique from computed X-ray tomography (CT) in which X-rays are transmitted from the X-ray tube through the patient to the detectors.
  - The term computed tomography indicates that slices through the body are generated by the computer aided **gamma camera.**
  - Cross-sectional images (CSI) allow the radiologists to focus on findings at a given section within the body. Besides, interference of overlying tissue is minimized.
  - Usually SPECT images are performed immediately after standard planar images (e.g. to evaluate further abnormalities in the spine as part of a bone scan) or as the primary procedure (e.g. for a BRAIN SCAN).

- **PET (Positron emission tomography).**
  - PET is a form of **nuclear medicine** that uses cyclotron–produced positron emitters and a special camera to detect them by virtue of the concurrent production of a pair of photons travelling away from each other at 180° after each positron undergoes an annihilation reaction.
  - PET is more advantageous than SPECT because the cyclotron can produce isotopes of carbon, oxygen and nitrogen–the recognised key elements of life.

> ***Note:*** *No isotopes of carbon (C), oxygen (O_2) and nitrogen (N_2) are suitable to standard nuclear gamma camera detection.*

  - The special requirements of PET scanning are balanced by the potential of actually following the biodistribution and fate of key molecules in many metabolic processes.

> ***Note :*** *PET is very expensive and so it is primarily a research tool. Even the most advanced nation of the world like USA has got this facility at a very limited specialised centres only.*

- **Recognised clinical uses of PET.**

i. Characterizing pulmonary nodules as benign (not active) vs. malignant (actively taking up a pharmaceutical like 18-fluorodeoxyglucose.

ii. Distinguishing between recurrent or residual brain tumor (metabolically active) and post-radiation therapy change (not metabolically active).

- The most commonly performed nuclear scan that is bone scan is sensitive to a wide variety of diseases including **osteomyelitis, primary and secondary bone tumours, arthritis, metabolic bone disease, trauma and avascular necrosis.**

> ***Note :*** *Currently two chief applications of bone scans are (a) detection of metastatic disease and (b) detection of osteomyelitis.*

- A **bone scan** is far more sensitive than plain films for detecting metastatic disease, except for **multiple myeloma**.
- Bone scan is highly sensitive for detecting early osteomyelitis and may precede plain film findings by a week or more.
- **Some common uses of renal scan includes:**
  a. To screen for renovascular hypertension (before and after an oral dose of an angiotensin–converting enzyme inhibitor (ACEI) e.g. **captopril**.
  b. To assess differential renal function (i.e. the exact GFR of each kidney), as in renal failure.
  c. To determine whether renal obstruction is present (frusemide) Lasix is given in the middle of the test and washes the pharmaceutical from a dilated but non-obstructed renal collecting system but does not wash out the pharmaceutical if true obstruction is present.
  d. To image the transplanted kidney.
- Lung scans are performed to rule out pulmonary embolism.

> ***Note :*** *Lung scans are useful to know differential ventilation in the lungs. For example, before pulmonary resection for a* ***primary lung tumour.***

- Cardiac ventriculogram, also called as MUGA (multigated acquisition) images the intracardiac blood pool during the cardiac cycle, using RBCs that have been tagged with radioactivity. Imaging may be done at rest or after excercise (stress). The cardiac ejection fraction is calculated this is most useful in patients undergoing chemotherapy to monitor cardiotoxicity.

> ***Note:*** *Other nuclear medicine done before and after exercise includes—*

a. A stress cardiac study (a test of myocardial perfusion).
The uptake of radiopharmaceutical in the myocardium is compared during rest and immediately after exercise. Areas of decreased uptake during both rest and exercise usually uptake during exercise only, with normal uptake at rest, usually represent areas experiencing exercise induced transient ischaemia.

- **WBC scans** reveal **"hot spots"** or areas of increased activity on the **gamma camera.** The primary uses of WBC scans are to detect areas of infection or abscess, especially when CT is equivocal or normal, and to detect osteomyelitis when three-phase bone scans are equivocal.
- **Gallium scans** are used because gallium is concentrated in areas of active infection or inflammation and in various tumours, especially in NHL. For the detection of abscess or infection, gallium has been largely replaced by radiolabelled leukocytes, but for lymphoma, especially to differentiate active residual disease from areas of scan, gallium remains quite useful.
- **Thyroid scan** is imaged to reveal hyperfunctioning and/or hypofunctioning areas such as nodules and masses. The study can establish that a clinically prominent gland is consistent with the diagnosis of Graves' disease (large, homogeneous, hyperfunctioning gland).

> ***Note:*** *Other condition, such as subacute thyroiditis (barely visible gland) and colloid goitre (large, inhomogeneous, irregular gland), also have typical imaging patterns.*

Traditionally, thyroid scanning has been applied to palpable nodules on the grounds that **"hot nodules"** are always benign (hyperfunctioning adenomas), whereas **"cold" nodules** may be nonfunctioning adenomas, cysts, or cancer.

> ***Note:*** *Recently, the trend has been to substitute FNAC/biopsy for thyroid scanning in the analysis of a single palpable thyroid nodule.*

- **Tc–99m** is the most commonly used nuclide in clinical practice. The most common uses of technetium includes:
  - i. Tc–99m–DTPA–a renal agent filtered by the glomeruli.
  - ii. Tc–99m–MAA–macroaggregated albumin used in the perfusion portion of the lung scan.
  - iii. Tc–99m–MDP (methylene diphosphonate)– the bone scan agent.
  - iv. TcO_4– (pertechnitate, a free state of technetium)– used for thyroid and testicular scans.
  - v. Tc–99m–Sestamibi–used for myocardial perfusion imaging.
- **Other radiopharmaceuticals used commonly in clinical practice**
  - i. I–131 (radioiodine) and I–123–used for thyroid imaging, I–131 is used for therapy of hyperthyroidism and thyroid C_A.
  - ii. Tl–201 (thallium)–used for myocardial perfusion imaging.
  - iii. In–111 (Indium)– used to tag WBCs.
- **New agents found clinical uses in nuclear medicine.**
  - a. A radiolabelled antibody marketed as "ONCOSCINT" is directed against the cell surface antigens of certain ovarian and colon CA. It has been available for a few years but has seen limited acceptance, largely because it is **very expensive.**
  - b. Similarly, a new brain imaging agents that cross the blood-brain barrier (BBB), producing superb images that reflect blood flow in the brain, have been limited acceptance because of the competition from MRI.
  - c. OCTREOTIDE, a somatostatin receptor agent, is the **newest agent.**

> **Note:** *It is used for imaging neuroendocrine tumours e.g.* ***carcinoid.***

- The I.V. radiopharmaceuticals imposes little anaphylaxis and the **radiational hazards** as compared to conventional X-rays are also very-very less. So, on the whole it is relatively a safer procedure as an diagnostic modality.

vi. *Radiographic Contrast Media (RCM)*

- RCM is intravenous contrast media injected during radiologic procedure to detect–
  a. Abnormal tissues (e.g.Tumour mass, inflammation) enhance differently than normal tissues with I.V. contrast; this enables the abnormal tissues to be identified and characterized.
  b. Contrast media opacify specific structures (e.g. blood vessels, the urinary tract) in order to detect abnormalities in them (e.g. filling defects, contour abnormalities).
- There are two types of iodinated contrast media.
  i. Ionic or HOCM (high osmolar contrast media).
  ii. Nonionic or LOCM (low osmolar contrast media).
- HOCM are composed of salts which dissociates into **cations** (sodium, meglumine) and **anions** (diatrizoate, iothalamate, and metrizoate).

> **Note:** *The osmolarity of HOCM is five times that of* ***serum***.

- LOCM are made up of monomers which are not salts hence do not dissociate.

> **Note:** *They are twice as much as the osmolarity of serum.*

- LOCM has fewer side-effects upon administration to HOCM. LOCM are less nephrotoxic than HOCM in patients with renal insufficiency.

- LOCM are about **five times more expansive than** HOCM. LOCM are **weak anticoagulants** than the HOCM.
- The major types of reactions to iodinated contrast media is—
  i. Anaphylactoid (idiosyncratic).
  ii. Non-idiosyncratic, and
  iii. Local reactions.

> ***Note:*** *All the 3 types can occur with both HOCM and LOCM.*

- **Anaphylactoid reactions**– These are so called anaphylactoid or idiosyncratic because the exact mechanism of action is unknown. These reactions occur unpredictably, although certain conditions increase the risk. The aetiology is probably multifactorial, involving the release of 5–HT (serotonine) and histamine, with resultant increased capillary permeability and constriction of bronchial smooth muscle cells.

> ***Note:*** *Anaphylactoid reactions include URTICARIA, FACIAL AND LARYNGEAL OEDEMA, BRONCHOSPASM and HYPOTENSION. Such reactions may be* ***life-threatening.***

- The **nonidiosyncratic reactions** to contrast media involve the direct effect of the contrast agent on an organ, e.g. nephrotoxicity, cardiac arrhythmias, myocardial ischemia, and vasovagal reactions.
- Local reactions to contrast media includes when contrast extravasates from the venous or arterial system into the adjacent soft tissues, in a small percentage of cases local **necrosis** may occur. This appears to occur more frequently with ionic than with nonionic contrast.

> ***Note:*** *Other types of local reactions include phlebitis secondary to endothelial damage following lower extremity* ***venography****.*

- The **reaction** may be categorized as **mild, moderate** or **severe.**

i. **Mild reaction** require no treatment, these includes HIVES.

ii. **Moderate reaction** require treatment but not life-threatening.

iii. **Severe reactions** are life-threatening and require immediate therapy. Most reactions occur within 20 meters of I.V. contrast administration.

> **Note:** *Delayed reactions are rare and usually require no treatment.*

Que. What distinguishes hypotension due to an idiosyncratic reaction from hypotension due to a vasovagal episode?

Ans. If the patient has **tachycardia**, it is likely that the cause is an anaphylactoid reaction. Patient experiencing a vasovagal reaction will be **bradycardic.**

> **Note:** *It is critical to distinguish the two conditions because the treatment for a vasovagal reaction is different from the treatment for an anaphylactoid reaction.*

- Those patients have hypotension with vasovagal episode should be treated with **ATROPINE** and **I.V.** FLUIDS.

> **Note:** *Those patient who are taking a b–blocker may experiencing an anaphylactoid reaction with bradycardia instead of tachycardia.*

- The overall incidence of contrast reactions for HOCM is about 5 to 12% and for LOCM is about 1 to 3%.
- **Conditions appear to increase the risk of a reaction to iodinated contrast media.**

> **Note:** *While some factors are controversial and based on anecdotal reports, some of the better–established risk factors includes–*

- Renal insufficiency.
- Bronchial asthma.
- Previous reaction to contrast media.

- Diabetes mellitus, when renal disease is present (elevated or raised CREATININE).
- Significant history of allergies.
- Severe cardiac or pulmonary disease.
- Very young and very old patients.

Note: *Less well established or controversial risk factors includes–*

- Phaeochromocytoma.
- Lupus.
- Myasthenia gravis.
- Hyperthyroidism.
- Multiple myeloma (especially if there is concurrent dehydration.)
- Sickle cell disease (iodinated contrast appears to promote sickling of erythrocytes).

Que: What is a typical premedication regimen before any contrast administration?

Ans:

i. **Prednisone** 50 mg orally 13, 5 and 1 hour before.

ii. **Diphenhydramine** 50 mg orally 1 hour before.

Side-effects include drowsiness due to medication.

- The incidence of fatal contrast reactions is approximately 1 per 100,000 administrations for both LOCM and HOCM.
- For myelography only nonionic contrast agents should be used.
- GADOLINIUM
- A rare, heavy–earth metal that when linked to ligands like DTPA, is used for I.V. contrast agent in MRI scan.
- Serious/lethal reactions with gadolinium is rare.
- **Gadolinium** is a **paramagnetic** agent that produces increased signal intensity on **T_1-weighted images.**

2

Radiophysics and Radiobiology

You Should Know

1. **Beta (β) rays** emitted from the nucleus of the atom result from disintegration of a neutron.
2. The purpose of inserting a **lead diaphragm** into the X-ray machine is to restrict the beam.
3. **Radium-226** is a naturally occurring radioactive element.
4. Characteristic radiation emitted from the **irradiated tissue** is totally absorbed in tissue.
5. Radiation doses to the occupational and non-occupational personnel are measured in unity of Rem.
6. The mininum wave length that can be obtained by the use of 60 KVP in an X-ray tube is about **0.20 A°.**
7. The **erythema dose** in conventional deep therapy unit is **650 rad.**
8. In view of the recent changes in uses of RBE and QF (Quality factor), QF is used solely for protection purposes.
9. **Linear energy transfer** (LET) for beta, gamma, X-rays having quality factor of 1-2 is 3.5 to 7 Kev per micron water (tissue).
10. **Dose equivalent** (DE) is defined as DE = rads × QF.
11. In the **energy balance of the emitted β particles,** the contribution of neutrino is that the energy of the neutrino is complementary to that of the β particles their sum being constant.

12. The fundamental difference between a **2 Mev van de Graff generator** and **200 KEV gamma** from a radioisotope in that the van de graff generator is **polychromatic** while the 200 Kev isotope is **monochromatic.**
13. In accurately measuring the surface dose of radiation in TELETHERAPY, the instrument used is **extrapolation chamber.**
14. In a **cyclotron,** electrons (β particles) cannot be accelerated.
15. In classical scattering, the **scattering radiation** has the same energy as the incoming beam.
16. When a pair is produced consisting of an electron and positron, the positron will recombine with one of the surrounding electrons, when the positron is at rest.
17. The **definition of roentgen** as a unit of quantity of X-ray or gamma radiation is valid up to 3 Mev.
18. When treating patients with a **cobalt-60 Teletherapy unit,** it is essential that a space of 15 to 20 cm be left between the diaphragm and the skin because secondary electrons from the diaphragm are stopped by this thickness of air and do not reach the patient.
19. In **Compton collisions,** the greater the energy of the incident photon the higher the energy of the recoil electron.
20. The **threshold energy for pair production** is 1.02 MEV of the incident photon. If this incident photon has an energy of 6 MEV. The most probable distribution of energy for each particle is positron 2.49 Mev, electron 2.49 Mev respectively.
21. Tumour-air ratio is defined as the ratio of the exposure dose at the tumour to the exposure dose at the tumour positioned in air. This ratio does not depend on the source skin distance.

***Note** : Tumour-air-ratio depends on:*
- *Depth of underlying tissue.*
- *The irradiated area.*
- *The quality of the beam.*

22. The isotope obtained upon disintegration of radium-226 that is a low energy β-emitter with a relatively long half-life used sometime back quite extensive for eye tumours is Radium-D.
23. **Materials of high Z** and usually of high density such as **salts of barium** and **iodine** are used as contrast media in diagnostic procedures because of their large photoelectric absorption. The K absorption edge of iodine and barium is approximately **30 Kev.**
24. In **stereoradiography** in order to get a proper three-dimensional effect, the ratio of the tube sift to the target film distance is equal to the ratio of the interpapillary distance to the viewing distance. For a chest radiograph taken at 72 inches, the tube shift should be 7.2 inches.
25. **ICRP recommends** that a diagnostic type of tube housing reduced the leakage radiation to at most **0.1/R/hr** at one meter from the target when the tube is operated continuously at the maximum rating.
26. In a **therapeutic type protective housing,** the leakage radiation shall be at most **1/R/hr** at one meter from the target.
27. For the **teletherapy units** at 1 meter in any direction from the source in the "off" position and maximum and average dose rates shall not exceed 10 m R/hr. and 2 m R/hr respectively.
28. The material used as **best filter for radiation** emitted from **Ra^{226}** is **gold.**
29. **Seven half-value layers** reduce the intensity of radiation to **0.78%.**
30. There are two spheres sphere 'A' with a diameter of 2 cm and sphere 'B' with a diameter of 3 cm. Both spheres are filled with Radon seeds with equal distribution per unit volume sphere 'B' received more radiation.
31. In the standard chest radiograph, the dose to the patients skin per exposure is approximately between 5 to 10 mR.
32. Background in a counter is largely due to **cosmic rays.**

33. The **decay factor** for any isotope depends, directly on the physical half-life.
34. During **fluoroscopy** the largest amount of scattered radiation originates in patients.
35. During **fluoroscopy** the safest position for the fluoroscopist is over the fluoroscopic screen.
36. The output on the table top of the fluoroscopic unit at 85 KVP and 5 MA shall not exceed 10s/minute.
37. Recognized **electromagnetic waves** are heat waves, infrared rays and radio waves.

Note: *Sound waves are not an electromagnetic waves.*

38. COMPTON effect depends on the number of electrons per gram of material.
39. In the **photoelectric effect,** the energy of the incoming radiation is given totally to the atom.
40. The best method for absolute determination of the absorbed dose is **calorimetry.**
41. The total absorbed dose of radiation from an **internal gamma emitter** depends on:
    - Concentration of the isotope.
    - Effective half-life.
    - K-factor: number of roentgens at 1 cm, from 1 cm of isotope.
42. The **4 parameters that define the quality** of a diagnostic film include:
    - Density.
    - Contrast.
    - Speed.
    - Latitude.
43. When to angled fields are directed through one side of a patient towards the tumour, it is very important that they should be aimed so that the intersection of their central lines lies below the tumour.
44. The **disadvantage of self-rectification in the X-ray tube** is possible danger of filament damage.
45. When the **accelerated electrons** in the tube strike the target to produce X-rays then approximately 1% of the energy of the electrons is converted into X-rays.

46. During radiographic exposure the **target film** distance is set at 36 inches and the object film distance is 3 inches. The percentage magnification is 9%.
47. Methods can used for the determination of the **spectral distribution of radiation** include:
    a. Absorption curve.
    b. Spectroscopy.
    c. Half-value layer.

> ***Note :*** *Law of Duane and Hunt cannot be used for the determinetion of the spectral distribution of radiation.*

48. The backscatter factors in **cobalt—60 Teletherapy** for large fields are about 5%.
49. **Accurate film dosimetry** can be used only in super voltage regions.
50. Methods used to remove **radioactive contamination** include:
    - Wasting with a detergent.
    - Treatment with dilute acids.
    - Soaking in non-radioactive solution of the contaminant.
51. It is advisable to wear **rubber gloves** when handling the urine of a patient who has received isotope treatment for thyroid C_A.
52. In " WIPE TESTS" performed on all radioactive sealed sources, the wipe sample must contain less than 0.005 vci activity to make the radioactive unit safe.
53. In **cobalt teletherapy** machines, the dose in the center of the field depends on the size of the irradiated field. This phenomenon is mostly due to scattering of the gamma (γ) photons from the walls of the collimator.
54. To achieve better than **99%** reliability in counting statistics, one must count within three standard deviation.
55. In a "SCINTILLATION COUNTER" the photomultiplier tube amplifies the current pulse by a factor of 1,000,000.

56. In TELEVISION CAMERAS, two types of pickup tubes, with different characteristics are used:

Vidicon Tube (V)	*Image Orthicon Tube (O)*
• Has lower sensitivity to light	• Has less radiation to the patient.
• Is less expensive and cheaper to operate	• Is not subject to log and smear.
• Is more resistant to shocks and temperature changes	• Is superior in the radiography of rapidly moving systems.
	• Signal to noise is very low at low signal levels.

57. **Internal conversions** and **electron capture** processes have no change in the atomic weight of the nucleus.
58. If the **biological half-life** of a particular isotope is 3 days and the effective half-life is 2 days, then the physical half life would be **six days.**
59. **Three phase** (TP) **circuits** are extensively used in producing a nearly constant potential for X-ray in diagnostic radiology. Compare the characteristics of a three phase circuit (TP) with those of single phase circuit (SP):

Three phase (TP) circuit	*Single phase (SP) circuit*
• Is more practical to transport and generate.	• Is less complicated in adjustment of the primary voltage.
• Supplies more power to X-ray tube per unit time.	• Is less complicated in starting and terminating of the exposure.
• The quality of radiation is harder.	• The intensity of radiation produced is smaller.
	• The efficiency of X-ray production is higher (lower heat losses).

60. In single hole collimator, the field of view increases on the distance from the collimator increases.

61. The sensitivity of the multihole focussed collimator with a large crystal is better than the sensitivity of the single hole collimator with a small crystal.
62. In the multihole focussed collimator with a large crystal and the single hole collimator with a small crystal, having the same hole diameter at the larger end, the spatial resolution of both is the same in the focal plane.
63. When a beam of photons all of the same energy enters the detecting crystal, a total absorption peak produces approximately the bell-shaped normal distribution. The resolution of the crystal is measured to be the full width at half-maximum peak in percentage of the peak energy (Kev).
64. All GEIGER-MUELLER TUBES operate in a region of voltage known as the plateau. A good G.M. tube should have a slope not greater than **5%.**
65. The **devices** contributed mostly to the development of SCINTILLATION COUNTERS is photomultiplier tube.
66. **Maximum permissible dose** (MPD) for occupational personnel exposed to ionizing radiation is **2.5 mR/hr.**
67. The absorption in tissue of fast neutrons is due mainly to direct collision of protons.
68. Number of atoms N present in different radionuclides having the same activity of 1 MCI depend on disintegration constant of the radionuclide.
69. The maximum energy ratings for X-ray tubes are usually expressed as rating charts to be used in X-ray exam of patients. These changer plotted as milliamperes versus maximum exposure time for different peak voltages.
70. The " BRAGG-GRAY THEORY" particularly useful in radiation **dosimetry** expresses mathematical relationship between ionization produced in the air cavity and the energy absorbed in the irradiated medium.

71. The law of "BUNSEN and ROSCOE" called the law of RECIPROCITY, states that the X-ray photographic effect depends only on the absorbed energy. This law of Reciprocity become invalid or fails when X-ray film is exposed within the intensifying cassette.
72. PROPORTIONAL COUNTER is a gas-filled detector operation in the intermediate voltage region. The most outstanding features of the proposition.
73. Following the process of electron conversion, there is a probability of emission of an AUGER ELECTRON from the atom. The auger electron is electron liberated from its orbit by the characteristic radiation within its own atom.
74. **Gamma (γ) ray** SPECTROMETER can be made to accept in many cases only the energies selected by the operator, and reject the scattered radiation. This selective process depends on likewise the higher the primary the better is the separation.
75. The typical value of the resolution of a sodium-iodide crystal is **8%.**
76. The action of ionizing radiation (excitation, ionization) is random, any atom with which it interacts is likely to be ionized.
77. Ions produced during irradiation can dissociated into **free radicals.**
78. Certain molecules, rare in number but highly important in function, are regarded as **key targets** for radiation in cells.
79. The relationship of survival of function to increasing dose radiation can indicate the number of molecules controlling the function.
80. Oxygen (O_2) enhances the magnitude of the radiation effect (an increase of 2 to 3 tissues).
81. The effect of O_2 is exerted at the time of energy exchange, probably by drawing radiation-produced free radicals into destructive auto-oxidative reactions.

82. The GENES are composed of macromolecules of DNA and **contain all the information** required for normal metabolism.
83. Exact duplication of each DNA macromolecule, before cell division permits the distribution of precisely the same genetic information from parent cell to its daughters.
84. The transfer of genetic material from one generation of individuals to the one that succeeds is accomplished through a process of cell division called **meiosis.**
85. **Mitosis** tends to preserve the status quo while **meiosis** lead towards genetic variation.
86. Exposure of population to **ionizing radiation** is detrimental to the population.
87. **Ionizing radiation** can either by direct or indirect action, break chromosomes. Such a break may restitute, causing no change, but on the other hand, structural rearrangement of chromosomes and even loss from cells to parts of as well as whole chromosomes may even following a break.
88. **Chromosome aberrations** are produced in many cell during radiation therapy and may occur following radiation exposure as part of diagnostic tests.
89. The **order of sensitivity of the vital organ systems to radiation,** progressing from the most sensitive to the most resistant, is the haematopoietic system, the gastrointestinal system and the CNS.
90. **Cataracts** occur after irradiation of the eyes, in particular with neutrons. It is not a common consequence of total body radiation.
91. The **biological effects of radiation** are dependent both on the kind as well as the quantity of radiation used.
92. **Relative biologic effectiveness** (RBE) depends on LET, but also upon the dose rate and upon whether the dose is given all at once or in fractions.

93. **Recovery from radiation exposure** may ensue, restoration of normal conditions depends on dose-rate as well as ion density.
94. The **immune response** consists of recognizing foreign material as foreign and removing it from the body.
95. Broadly foreign materials are grouped into 3 categories: (I) viruses and cells (II) groups or cells/tissues (tissues or organs) and (III) non-living materials like chemicals and toxins, etc.
96. The **repair of sublethal radiation injury** by cells depends on—
    - The dose of radiation.
    - The fractionation.
    - The dose rate.
97. The BERGONIE-TRIBONDEAU LAW was formulated in 1905. This law is based on clinical and pathological observation relates to radiosensitivity and cellular differentiation.
98. **X-rays are produced** when a fast moving swarm of electrons are suddenly decelerated by anode placed in its path of a cathode ray or X-ray tube.

> ***Note:*** *The ANODE of X-ray tube is made up of TUNGSTEN with atomic number of 74 and melting point of 3370° C.*

99. KVP determines the maximum energy produced by the X-ray.
100. **X-ray** is nothing but a **electromagnetic wave** with wave length of 1/10,000 of light.
101. RADIOGRAPHY is based on differential absorption of **X rays.**

> ***Note:*** *Dense tissues like bone absorb X-rays more readily than soft tissues.*

102. Structures not penetrated by X-rays become RADIOPAQUE whereas those penetrated become RADIOLUCENT.
103. **X-ray film** consists of **cellulose acetate** coated on both sides with silver bromide 0.001 inch thick.

104. In standard **X-ray filmography** radiopaque structures produce **white shadow** while radiolucent produce or cost **black shadow.**
105. It has been seen that when X-rays strike certain metallic salts (Zinc cadmium sulphide), the rays make them to fluoresce. This phenomenon is called **fluorescence** and its principle is used in FLUOROSCOPY.
106. **High voltage (energy) machines** produce better X-ray picture with less exposure time while low energy machines with long exposure time make patient vulnerable for receiving more radiation.
107. Developer solution contains METOL, anhydrous sodium sulphite whereas FIXER solution contains sodium thiosulphate, potassium metasulphite and ammonium chloride.
108. The main function of developing is to reduce the expose silver halide crystal to metallic silver without harming unexposed silver halide crystals. It contains **4 essential ingradients.**
    a. Organic reducing agents–a mix. of hydroquinone and metol.

    > ***Note :*** *Hydroquinone provides contrast while metol gives finer detail.*

    b. Activator–Na_2CO_3 and NaOH is used.
    c. Restrainer–KBr and KI–Antifogging agent.
    d. Preservative–Sodium sulfite.
109. The two most important factors in development include:
    - The temperature of the developing solution (optimum 20 to 22°C).
    - The total time of development.
110. **Fixing solution** consits of 4 essential ingrediants like **Fixing agents** (hypo), **preservative** (sodium sulfite), **Hardner** (chrome alum, potash alum) and **Acid** (H_2SO_4 or acetic acid).
111. **Rapid fixer:** contains in addition NH_4Cl. (ammonium chloride) and thereby reduces the

fixing time to half. A satisfactory fixer requires about 1 to 4 minutes to clear a film.

Note: *A fixer is said to be exhausted if the fixing time is prolonged beyond 10 minutes.*

112. **Film badge** or **Dosimeter** is used to measure radiation exposure.
113. **X-ray film become darker** owing to over exposure, high temperature of developer, longer development time, etc.
114. **Faint image** (weak) is due to under exposure, old developer at low temperature, short development time, highly concentrated developer.
115. The direction of eddy current is given by **Lenz's law.**
116. **Eddy currents** are used to produce **magnetic brakes.**
117. **X-ray therapy tubes** operate at low MA values of tube current to provide X-rays of four main KV energy ranges.
    - Low voltage 50 to 120 KV.
    - Intermediate voltage 130 to 150 KV.
    - Orthovoltage 160 to 300 KV.
    - Mega/Super voltage 4 MV or more.

3

Neuroradiology

You Should Know

1. Basilar invagination or Basilar impression is encountered in **Paget's disease.**
2. In Basilar impression, the tip of the odontoid process is above CHAMBERLAIN'S or MACGREGOR'S LINE by a distance of 5 mm.
3. **Suture widening** as a manifestation of increased intracranial pressure (ICP) is seen most frequently below the age of 12 years.
4. The **basal angle** is formed by two lines having an apex at the TUBERCULUM SELLAE.
5. The average size of the **basal angle** is **134°.**
6. A **basal angle** greater than **143°** indicates PLATYBASIA.
7. **Calcification of the pineal body** is encountered in 55% of adults over 20 years of age.
8. The habenular calcification is located about 5 mm anterior to the pineal gland.
9. Premature closure of the CORONAL SUTURE results in **brachycephaly.**
10. Premature closure of the SAGITTAL SUTURE results in→ **dolichocephaly.**
11. The earliest radiologic evidence of increased ICP affecting the sella turcica can be observed on the anterior cortical bone at the base of the **dorsum sellae.**
12. Approximately 5 to 10% of CHROMOPHOBE PITUITARY ADENOMAS fail to produce any enlargement of the pituitary fossa.

13. Calcifications within a CRANIOPHARY-NGIOMA is encountered in approximately **70%** of cases.
14. **Tumours of the 8th nerve** affecting the petrous pyramid most frequently involve the meatus of the internal auditory canal.
15. The upper limits of normal for the vertical measurement of the meatal portion of the internal auditory canal are **8 mm.**
16. With radiograph using a 30 to 40 inch target film distance the **optic foramen** should not exceed a measurement of **6.5 mm.**
17. Optic nerve gliomas are seen in combination with → VON RECLINGHOUSEN DISEASE OR NEUROFIBROMATOSIS.
18. **Optic nerve gliomas** are most frequently encounted in children below the age of 15 years.
19. A clear area of bone destruction that is surrounded by a very sharply delimited margin of increased density is descriptive of an EPIDERMOID tumour.
20. **Calcification** is encountered in **chordomas** in **33%** of cases.
21. The most frequent site for intracranial MENINGIOMAS is the **frontal parasagittal sinus.**
22. Plain film **signs of meningioma** include tumour calcification and incrased vascularity.
23. One of the signs of MENINGIOMA on the plain film is → **enlargement of the foramen spinosum.**
24. **Tumour calcification** is encountered in meningiomas in **10 to 20%** of cases.
25. **Parallel tracks of intracranial calcification** are encountered in → VENOUS ANGIOMA.
26. **Multiple scattered intracranial calcifications** are seen with → TUBEROUS SCLEROSIS.
27. In the STURGE-WEBER SYNDROME, the cerebral involvement is most frequently encountered in the **occipital lobe.**

28. HABE NULAR calcification usually takes the configuration of the ROMAN letter → "C".
29. A glioma with an incidence of calcification of more than **50%** is an **oligodendroglioma.**
30. **Cytomegalic inclusion disease** is associated with calcification in the distribution of periventricular.
31. In PNEUMOENCEPHALOGRAPHY, the tips of the temporal horns may show improved visualization with the forward Sumersault maneuver.
32. The maximum distance on pneumoencephalography from the dorsum sellae to the floor of the fourth venticle is → **4.0 cm.**
33. **Twining's line** is used to determine the position of the 4th ventricle.
34. A condition described by **Dandy and Walker** includes atresia of the formina Luschka and Magendie.
35. The pituitary adenoma accounts for approximately 1/5th fraction of all brain tumours.
36. The EPENDYMOMA occurs most frequently in the → **4th ventricle.**
37. A **colloid cyst** is a tumour mass which occurs in the anterior portion of the 3rd ventricle.
38. The PINEALOMA presents as a mass projecting into the posterior portion of the 3rd ventricle.
39. On PNEUMOENCEPHALOGRAPHY, hemisphere mass lesions producing an angular shift in which the top of the septum pellucidum is displaced more than the base are usually located above the transverse plane of the foramen of Monro.
40. On **pneumoencephalography** with hemispheric mass lesions, a curved shift of the septum pellucidum and 3rd ventricle is encountered in lesions below the transverse plane of the foramen of Monro.
41. The most frequent cerebellar neoplasm of adult life is the → HAEMANGIOBLASTOMA.

42. Angulation and forward displacement of the aqueduct of Sylvius is characteristic of masses affecting the → Cerebellar hemisphere.
43. Cerebellopontine angle masses cause contralateral and posterior displacement of the aqueduct and 4th ventricle.
44. The suprasellar extent of a pituitary tumour is usually determined by the involvement of the anterior inferior portion of the 3rd ventricle.
45. Focal enlargement of the spinal canal in the thoracic lumbar region associated with a central filling defect on myelography is characteristic of → DIASTEMATOMYELIA.
46. **Pyogenic infection of the spinal canal** is most likely to cause on myelography an extradural deformity located dorsally.
47. **Spinal canal masses** that displace the spinal cord and compress and obliterate the subarachnoid space are located extradurally.
48. A **fusiform enlargement of the spinal cord** in the cervical or thoracic region is most likely due to a **glioma.**
49. The range of normal for the transverse diameter of the cervical cord in the cervical and thoracic area as a percent of the spinal canal is → **50 to 75%.**
50. The **critical sagittal diameter of the spinal canal** with regard to the presence of neurologic signs due to spondylosis deformans is **less than 13 mm.**
51. The normal **carotid angiogram**–arterial phase–lasts approximately **1.0 to 2.5 seconds.**
52. The "TRAM-TRACK" appearance seen on carotial angiography represents a fistula between the middle meningeal artery and paired veins.
53. Early venous filling in cranial angiography usually indicates a tumour or an A-V malformation.
54. **After evacuation of a subdural haematoma,** the displaced middle structures return to midline usually in about 2 to 4 weeks.

55. **Circulation time in carotid angiography** is defined as the time from maximum concentration of the contrast substance in the carotid siphon to maximum concentration of the contrast substance in the parietal veins.
56. EPIDURAL HAEMATOMAS may result from a tear in the middle meningeal anterior dural artery, parasagittal veins, transverse sinus and arachnoid granulations.
57. **Glioblastoma multiforme** (Astrocytoma grade III or IV) is avascular on cerebral angiography in approximately 12 to 15% of cases.
58. **Meningiomas** are avascular on cerebral angiography in approximately **30 to 40%** of cases.
59. The **nerve closest to the cavernous carotid artery** is the **abducent N** or **6th cranial nerve** (CN).
60. The commonest cause of a caroticocavernous fistula is trauma.
61. **Craniopharyngiomas** and **chromophobe adenoma** both may present as suprasellar masses. The sign that would make the diagnosis of chromophobe almost certain is tumour vessels.
62. The LENTICULO–STRIATE ARTERIES are of value in localizing small deep frontal masses.
63. While not invariable so, a semilunar extracerebral zone on cerebral angiography usually indicates **acute subdural haematoma.**
64. A cerebral abscess may have a vascular wall. This appears usually in the **venous phase.**
65. **Mycotic aneurysms** have a propensity to distribute in the **middle cerebral artery.**
66. On **carotid angiography,** with a selective internal carotid injection, one would expect the posterior communicating artery and the posterior cerebral artery to fill in approximately **50%** of cases.
67. The **anterior choroidal artery** supplies the choroid plexus of the lateral ventricle, the hippocampus, and the basal ganglia.

68. The **angiographic Sylvian point** on cerebral angiography represents the most posterior point of the Sylvian fissure.
69. The **paired posterior inferior cerebellar arteries** are symmetrical in approximately 25% of cases.
70. UNCAL HERNIATION with resultant pressure on the brainstem may cause death by arterial and/or venous haemorrhage of brainstem vessels.
71. The **left common carotid artery** originates from the innominate artery in approximately **6 to 9%** of cases.
72. **Post-traumatic occlusion of the middle cerebral artery** usually occurs 24 to 48 hours after trauma.
73. The artery of BERNASCONI and CASSINARI is most apt to supply a tentorial tumour.
74. Azygous anterior cerebral artery occurs in MONKEYS.
75. Spasm in subarachnoid cerebral haemorrhage after aneurysm rupture has been shown to be most intense in the first 2–3 days.
76. Heart failure in infancy of **"high output"** type is occasionally found to be due to aneurysm of the **great vein of Galen.**
77. In an SOL of the thalamus, one might expect to see changes in the venous phase of the lateral cerebral angiogram such as elevation of the thalamo–striate vein.
78. The clino–parietal line in adults is a good landmark. The middle cerebral artery (main branches) should fall not more than 1.0 cm above this line.
79. **"Draping"** of temporal lobe vessels usually indicates that the mass is **intracerebral.**
80. The most common persistent carotid basilar anastomosis is the → HYPOGLOSSAL artery.
81. The internal cerebral vein is located in the cistern of the velum interpositum.

82. The left vertebral artery arises directly from the arch in 12 to 15% of cases.
83. The most common location of an epidural haematoma is the **middle fossa.**
84. The veins of the posterior fossa drain into the galenic system, petrosal sinuses, and the trocular and neighboring dural sinuses.
85. Anterior choroidal artery has its origin immediately above the posterior communicating artery.
86. A disparity between the curve of the pericallosal artery (wide sweep) on the lateral projection and the actual size of the lateral ventricle as demonstrated by the thalamo-striate vein in the **half-axial view** is suggestive of a mass in the corpus callosum.
87. aneurysms of the middle meningeal artery are usually **false aneurysms.**
88. In direct puncture **vertebral angiography,** one would expect to visualize the anterior spinal artery in approximately **50%** of cases.
89. In the case of **multiple cerebral aneurysms** with a **subarachnoid haemorrhage,** the one that most likely to bleed is the largest aneurysm.
90. Each carotid artery carries approximately 300 cc blood per minute.
91. Cerebral and cortical atrophy on **cerebral angiography** will appear as dilated ventricles with an avascular extracerebral zone.
92. An **avascular temporal lobe mass,** biopsied, shows intracellular inclusion bodies. The most likely aetiology is **Herpes simplex virus.**
93. Increase in partial CO_2 in man causes dilatation of → **cerebral arteries.**
94. The CORPUS CALLOSUM is involved in glioblastoma multiforme (ASTROCYTOMA GRADE III or IV) in approximately 33% of cases.
95. The cerebral veins dilate during **cerebral angiography.**

96. **Hemiatrophy of the brain** may have the following skull changes:
    - Thickened cranial vault.
    - Elevation of the petrous ridge.
    - Excessive pneumatization of the temporal bone.
97. **Leptomeningeal cyst** is associated with a fracture with tearing of the dura.
98. **Exophthalmos** is associated most frequently with **neurofibromatosis.**
99. The most helpful examination in the diagnosis of **optic nerve glioma** is pneumoencephalography.
100. The A-1 segment of the anterior cerebral artery is atretic in 25%.
101. Displacement of the Sylvian triangle forwards indicates a mass in **occipital regions.**
102. **Arteriovenous malformations** account for 2% of sub-arachnoid haemorrhages.
103. **Secondary cranial synostosis** is not seen in vitamin 'C' deficiency.
104. The average volume of the adult lateral ventricles is **20 ml.**
105. **Herniation of the anterior part of the hippocampus** is demonstrated by medial displacement of anterior choroidal artery.
106. **Herniation of intervertebral discs** is seen least frequently at the T_{3-4} level.
107. **Pneumographic signs of atrophy (brain)** may be seen 10 days after head injury.
108. To better demonstrate a **right frontal subdural haematoma** by right carotid arteriography, the patient's head should be turned towards the side of the injection.
109. Opening of the supratonsillar loop of the posterior inferior cerebellar artery on the lateral view indicates fourth ventricular tumour.
110. Lateral displacement of both lateral mesencephalic veins indicate a brainstem tumour.

111. The ARNOLD CHIARI MALFORMATION involves downward herniation of cerebellar tissue.
112. Frequently seen in TUBEROUS SCLEROSIS is filling defects of the **lateral ventricle.**
113. Primary CNS tumours commonly metastasize through the CSF to cause leptomeningeal seeding or **DROP METASTASES** include:
   - Medulloblastomas.
   - Ependymomas.
   - Primitive neuroectodermal tumours (PNET) and pineal tumours.
   - Malignant gliomas.

> ***Note** : The diagnosis of leptomeningeal seeding is definitively made by CSF cytology. Gadolinium enhanced MRI of the neuraxis is useful and NON-INVASIVE but is less sensitive than CSF cytology.*

114. The most common **tumour found in the cerebellopontine angle** includes:
   - Acoustic neuromas.
   - Metastatic tumours.
   - Meningiomas.
   - Epidermoid tumours.
115. **Bilateral Acoustic Neuromas** are diagnostic of NEUROFIBROMATOSIS type II.
116. The syndrome associated with cerebellar and spinal haemangioblastomas is VON HIPPEL LINDAU SYNDROME (VHLS).
117. A hormonally active most common pituitary adenoma is **prolactinoma.**
118. The gold standard to diagnose carotid stenosis is **selective carotid angiography.**
119. Fibromuscular dysplasia demonstrates irregularity and **"stack of coins"** characteristic of a vasculitis.
120. The most common locations for a hypertensive haemorrhage is the **basal ganglia** (especially the putamen), the thalamus, the pons, the cerebellum and the subcortical white matter.

121. The most common cause of recurrent intracranial haematomas in the elderly is AMYLOID ANGIOPATHY stained by **congored.**
122. The common cuases of **subarachnoid haemorrhage** (SAH) include:
    - Rupture of a "berry" aneurysm (the most common cause).
    - Trauma.
    - Hypertension.
    - Coagulopathy.
    - Dural A-V malformation.

    Note: *diagnosis of SHA is made by CAT scan or LP.* (applies to: Trauma, Hypertension, Coagulopathy, Dural A-V malformation)
123. The Berry aneurysms are most commonly located at the middle cerebral arterial bifurcation. Angiography remains the gold standard in the diagnosis of ruptured berry aneurysm.
124. HSV type I is the commonest aetiologic agent encephalitis in older children and adults while HSV–II is seen in infants.

> ***Note:*** *For diagnosing encephalitis MRI is more sensitive than CAT scan.*

125. MRI is much more sensitive than CAT scan in diagnosing MULTIPLE SCLEROSIS.

4

Radiology of Paranasal Sinuses, Orbits, Temporal Bones, Larynx and Pharynx

You Should Know

1. A complete examination of the sinuses should include prone PA **(Caldwell)**, erect **Water's** and an erect lateral plus a prone open mouth Water's and a prone base.
2. An optimal Caldwell PA view projects the petrous ridge as the level of the inferior orbital rim to give a clear view of the paper plate and the orbital floor (or antral roof).
3. A **proper lateral view** is obtained as follows : Erect with sagittal plane rotated 5° toward film.
4. **Maxillary sinusitis** will often show radiologically complete opacification due to thickened membrane with or without a fluid level indicating secretion.
5. A **dense antrum** can be caused by a post-operative Caldwell Luc antrostomy with removal of mucosal lining with resultant sclerosis of the antral wall and a decrease in size of the sinus.
6. Unilateral pain in the frontal, supraorbital, retrobulbar, temporal, vertex and occipital regions without a stiff neck is often due to **sphenoidal sinusitis.**
7. **Frontal, maxillary** and **sphenoid sinusitis** are readily diagnosed by proper technique and require similar principles in diagnostic evaluation, being air-containing cavities of variable diameters and with walls of variable thickness.

8. **Retention cysts** occur most commonly in the antra and occur rarely on the antronasal wall mimicking an antral poly which arises near the orifice and may hang downward may block the antrum marking it opaque and may extrude into the nasopharynx as a choanal polyp.
9. **Retention cysts** ensue most commonly in the antra and occur on the roof, lateral wall and the floor. Occasionally they expand and cause **mucocele formation** paradoxically leading to enophthalmos.
10. **Retention cysts** occur most commonly in the antrum and can mimic mucosal swelling on the floor of the antrum caused by a **periapical dental abscess.**
11. A "TRIPOD–FRACTURE" is better considered a "quadripod fracture" because it involves four sites:
    - The hypomaticofrontal suture.
    - The inferior orbital rim.
    - The lateral wall of maxillary sinus.
    - The zygomatic arch.
12. **Retention cysts** occur most commonly in the antrum and can resemble a blow out fracture of the floor of the orbit except for the absence of fracture lines.
13. For practical purposes facial bone laminography, as in other parts of the body, best done in these two positions because of ease of performance and interpretation is AP (face up) and lateral views.
14. Ethmoid sinusitis shows a unilaterally dense ethmoid labyrinth, rarely with bone destruction and occasionally extending to the orbit producing increased orbital density due to cellulitis.
15. Regarding an ethmoid fracture is–
    - A type of orbital blowout fracture.
    - Frequently associated with periorbital emphysema.

- Clinically manifested by epistaxis and periorbital ecchymosis.
- Easily seen on laminograms as well as a Caldwell, Water's and optic foramen view.

16. Regarding **dental films**—
    - Give good detail of the alveolar ridge in suspected carcinoma.
    - Are routinely used in unilateral maxillary sinusitis whether clinically suspected or radiographically diagnosed.
    - May be used under the cheek to show parotid duct calculi
    - Of the upper alveolar ridge are routine in inflammatory swelling of the cheek.
17. Regarding an **anterior cranial fossa fracture with cerebrospinal rhinorrhoea**—
    - May not be seen radiologically but the evaluation begins here.
    - If present, will be diagnosed by observing cotton packing in the nose fluoresce with a Wood's light after introducing fluorescein by L.P.
    - Should be suspected in all nasion fractures.
    - May only be recognized on an optic foramen view.
18. Regarding **sinus malignancy**—
    - Usually fills the sinus and destroy bone.
    - Can be mimicked by Wegener's granulomatosis and mucormycosis.
    - Is rare in the sphenoid.
    - May be studied by laminography.
19. Regarding antral carcinoma—
    - Is reasonably common and readily diagnosed correctly.
    - May destroy the alveolar ridge.
    - May invade the orbit.
    - May extend to the middle fossa by perineural or direct extension.
20. Regarding **juvenile angiofibromas**—
    - Typically arise more anteriorly than adenoid.

- Frequenly extend into the pterygomaxillary fissure.
- May erode the floor of the sphenoid sinus and even invade the orbit and the anterior and middle fossae.
- Angiography is helpful.

21. The normal lateral view of the nasopharynx shows the distance from the tangent of the eustachian tube orifice to the tangent of the nasopharyngeal vault of the nasopharynx to be about 10 mm and readily seen using proper technique.
22. Regarding a **nasopharyneal neoplasm**—
    - Can involve all cranial nerves.
    - Should be suspected with epistaxis, headaches and ipsilateral 6th CN palsy.
    - May destroy the petrous apex.
    - Shows a good response to radiation therapy if recognized before cranial nerve involvement, bone destruction or metastasis.
23. The commonest metastatic sinus cancer is kidney.
24. The **optic foramen view** shows the foramen to be properly projected when seen at the inferolateral aspect of the orbital rim at 4:30 and 7:30.
25. An **orbital blowout fracture** involving ethmoid and orbital floor is best seen on **Caldwell's view.**
26. The **diagnostic accuracy of orbital blowout fracture** diagnosis by plain films and laminography would be cent percent (100%).
27. A diagnostic **intraocular foreign body** evaluation is best done by—
    - Scout films consisting of Caldwell and lateral.
    - Lateral views with the patient looking up, down and straight ahead.
    - A bone free dental film if possible.
    - Sweet's or other specific localization procedures.
28. The **inferior orbital fissure** can be seen on—
    - The Caldwell view.

- Stenver's view.
- The basal view.
- Lateral laminograms.

29. The **inferior orbital fissure** is involved in all zygomaticomaxillary complex fractures.
30. ORBITAL VENOGRAPHY finds its chief use in an orbital varix suspect.
31. ORBITAL ARTERIOGRAPHY is best used for A-V shunts and meningiomas.
32. Regarding **optic nerve glioma**—
    - May be congenital.
    - Is usually seen on optic foramen views.
    - May erode the optic canal in its intracranial canalicular or intraorbital portion such that pluridirectional laminography is needed for accurate assessment.
    - Can be recognized by retrobulbar contrast study.
33. The commonest tumour causing unilateral exophthalmos is ANGIOMA.
34. Regarding **orbital tumours**—
    - There may be fairly specific radiologic characteristic as in—
      i. Eosinophilic granulomatous bone destruction.
      ii. Dermoids involving bone.
      iii. Sphenoid ridge meningiomas.
    - Angiography, contrast orbitography with or without laminography and ultrasound may be involved.
    - Orbital enlargement is common in infants and children but less so in an adult.
    - Metastases are to be considered both to the soft tissues and the bones of the orbits.
35. Primary EPIDERMOIDS cause a fairly typical lucent defect with a sclerotic, often lobulated, margin.
36. Regarding FIBROUS DYSPLASIA—
    - Can constrict the **orbit** and **optic** canals on occasion.

- Becomes **malignant** on occasion.
- Continues into adult life.
- Shows lucent areas.
- Usually involves more than one bone.

37. Orbital cellulitis can be mistaken for a periapical abscess with cellulitis spreading from the cheek to the orbit.

> ***Note** : Dental films will be helpful here.*

38. The mastoid process is best seen on **lateral oblique view**.
39. Fractures of the temporal bone are of two basic types linear (axial) and transverse.
40. A **linear fracture of the temporal bone** is usually referred to as a **basal skull fracture,** presenting with bleeding from the involved ear and may show subcutaneous haemorrhage over the mastoid process–"BATTLE'S SIGN". It is best seen on a **Schüller** or **temporomandibular joint view.**
41. A **transverse fracture** is transverse or perpendicular to the axis of the temporal bone and often **transects** the **7th** (facial) and **8th** (vestibulocochlear) **nerves** (CN).
42. **Acoustic nerve tumours** usually arise from the vestibular division laterally and may erode the falciform crest.
43. **Acoustic nerve tumours** usually arise in the cerebellopontine angle and are well evaluated by **laminography.**
44. **Paget's disease of the temporal bone** resembles Paget's disease of bone elsewhere.
45. Regarding GLOMUS TUMOURS—
    - Derive their blood supply chiefly from the **external carotid.**
    - Should be routinely studied by **retrograde jugular venography** as the intravascular component of these tumours cannot otherwise be demonstrated ideally preoperatively.

- May be difficult to see destruction on the occipital projection but show well on AP **laminography.**
- **Schüller views** may help show jugular destruction.
- May be well seen on a **water's type projection** with the petrous bones projecting through the open mouth.

46. Regarding **linear tomography**—
    - Elongates structures running in the axis of travel.
    - Shows the internal auditory canal very well.
    - Shows the jugular foramina well.
    - Can show ossicular destruction and associated scutal, attic, and antral destruction.
47. **Cholesteatoma formation** in chronic otitis is usually seen in—
    - Schuller's view.
    - Owen's view.
    - Base view on occasion.
    - Law's view or lateral oblique view if destruction is extensive enough.
48. **Otosclerosis of the cochlea** is readily seen on **pluridirectional laminography**.
49. Regarding NASOPHARYNGEAL tumours—
    - Have a high incidence among some orientals.
    - EBV may be associated causative agent.
    - May destroy the skull base in the petrosphenoidal region.
    - Can present with a serous otitis secondary to eustachian tube blockage.
    - May be associated with an isolated 6th (Abducent) N palsy and epistaxis.
    - If discovered early responds well to radiotherapy.
50. Among some other lesions involving the **cerebellopontine angle** or **temporal bone** than acoustic nerve tumours include—
    - Metastatic renal cell C_A in Von-Hippel Lindau's syndrome (VHLS).

- Fibrous dysplasia.
- Reparative granuloma.
- Wegener's granuloma.

51. An ideal lateral film of the neck is made as follows, the chin is elevated. The deltoid touches a 10 × 12 cassette with the patient in true lateral position. The patient then rotates the sagittal plane by turning the face 5° towards the cassette. The film is taken while the patient is breathing in quietly. The cervical spine is seen adequately to evaluate any important abnormality.
52. Regarding **laminography**—
    - **AP laminography** is comfortable for the patient. Positioning is easier. A preliminary lateral across the table film is advisable to ascertain the axis of the ventricle. If this axis is not perpendicular to the table top, the true and false cord thickness and ventricular size. Films are done from skin surface to the level of the cervical spine at 0.5 cm intervals. A falsetto "e" or "o" and inspiratory phonation may be used. The advantage of the procedure is that it is the scope of the armamentarium of a well-instructed technician freeing the radiologist for consultations about 30 minutes is enough time to allot.
53. Regarding **laryngeal fluoroscopy**—
    - Following the acquisition of all appropriate clinical information one can safely say that he has performed a complete study of the laryngopharynx by a lateral soft tissue film, image amplified laryngeal and chest fluoroscopy, barium swallow, laminograms and a laryngogram.
54. Regarding contrast laryngography—
    - Air or spontaneously aspirated contrast such as barium, watery contrast (Gastrografin) or oily contrast (Lipidol or Dionosil) or purposefully induced contrast using oily Dionsil are the many types of contrast study available in clinical practice.

> ***Note :*** *Many times air contrast could be used because of its safety and reliability e.g. in the trachea.*

55. The lesion might be anticipated from a soft tissue lateral neck film is **laryngeal C_A** involving the anterior commissure with subglottic extension.
56. Regarding **nasal cycle** (NC)—
    - During nasal cycle (NC), the mucosa of the middle and inferior turbinate swells on one side, while the other side constricts. It is seen in each individual and its length varies from **30 minutes to 7 hours.** The imaging correlate of the NC is asymmetry of the thickness of the turbinates on CT scan.

> ***Note :*** *In contrast to findings in acute rhinitis, the swollen side never occludes the nasal cavity and should be recognized as a normal finding.*

57. CT is indicated for **acute sinusitis** in cases of suspected complications, when surgical drainage is planned and when the diagnosis is uncertain.
58. Patients with recurrent acute or chronic sinusitis that is incompletely controlled by medical therapy may be candidates for **functional endoscopic sinus surgery** (FESS). CT plays a critical role in evaluating these patients as the exact location and extent of disease is shown. CAT also reveals anatomic variations that predispose patients to develop sinusitis. These variations must be identified preoperatively to avoid surgical complications. CT is also indicated if the diagnosis of chronic sinusitis is uncertain.
59. The **role of MRI scan in the evaluation of sinusitis** is limited. While CT reveals detailed bony anatomy, no signal on MRI scan can be produced by cortical bone.
60. **MRI scan is the investigation of choice** for evaluation of intracranial complications of sinusitis and to distinguish inflammatory from neoplastic disease within the sinuses.

61. Regarding **ostiomeatal unit** (OMU)—
   - OMU is a complex drainage pathway of the maxillary, anterior ethmoid and frontal sinuses into the middle nasal meatus.

> ***Note :*** *Recognized components of the OMU include the uncinate plate, inner maxillary sinus ostium, infundibulum, semilunar hiatus, middle turbinate, middle nasal meatus and the ethmoidal bulla.*

62. The OMU should always be imaged in the direct coronal plate on CAT scan (3 mm slice).

> ***Note :*** *If a patient cannot tolerate neck extension, 1 mm contiguous images can be obtained on a helical CT scanner and coronal images can be reconstructed from the imaging data set.*

63. Regarding **functional endoscopic sinus surgery** (FESS)—
   - A relatively recently developed but now widely accepted surgical technique during which a set of rigid, fiberoptic endoscopes is used to examine the nasal and sinus cavities. Various specialized instruments are inserted alongside the viewing endoscope.

> ***Note :*** *FESS has essentially replaced external procedures that were used for surgical treatment of sinusitis.*

64. The **concept of FESS** is to treat chronic or recurrent acute sinusitis by restoring normal physiology.
65. A **"Haller cell"** is an air cell found in the bone of orbital floor.

> ***Note :*** *It is formed by progressive inferior pneumatization of the anterior ethmoid into the orbital floor.*

66. A **"Concha bullosa cell"** is an air cell that has formed within the middle nasal turbinate. If ostium is not identified on CT scan.

> ***Note :*** *A concha bullosa may interfere with air flow through the middle meatus and may adversely affect OMU drainage.*

67. An "**Agger nasi cell**" is the most anterior of all the anterior ethmoid air cells. Although it has a separate embryologic origin, it can be thought of as an air cell in the lacrimal bone, occasionally pneumatizing into the orbital plate of the ethmoid (lamina papyracea).

> ***Note :*** *A large agger nasi cell may form the floor of the frontal recess.*

68. An "**Onodi Cell**" is a posterior ethmoidal air cell that has extended posteriorly to pneumatize the **planum sphenoidale.** The importance of this anatomic variationis that it results in a posterior ethmoid air cell bordering the optic canal, instead of the sphenoid sinus.

> ***Note :*** *Posterior ethmoid disease in patients with an Onodi cell may therefore affect the optic nerve; the optic nerve can be injured during posterior ethmoidectomy in such individuals.*

69. Regarding the imaging feature of **sinonasal polyps.**
    - Sinonasal polyps may be single, multiple, or diffuse. All polyps are oedematous and are therefore low in density on CT, low in signal intensity on T_1-weighted MR and hyper-intense on T_2-weighted MRI.

> ***Note :*** *Polyps are seen as smooth soft–tissue masses in the nasal cavity, which are most commonly seen in middle meatus. They tend to elongate inferiorly and "drip" downward. An isolated sinus polyp is less frequent, producing a rounded or pedunculated soft tissue mass in a sinus cavity.*

70. Regarding the imaging feature of **diffuse sinonasal polyps.**
    - In diffuse polyposis, there are numerous polyps throughout the nose and involved sinus

cavities. The pressure of these polyps may affect the surrounding bony structures with widening of the nasal cavities with splaying of the lateral nasal walls and expansion of involved air cells. There is severe impairment of sinus drainage. Secretions are entrapped and become dessicated, which on CAT scan produces high attenuation material that insinuates between and around the individual low density polyps.

71. Regarding **mucocele:**
    - A mucocele produces expansion of a sinus cavity.
    - Mucoceles are low in density on CAT scan. Protein content and hydration status affect the signal intensity pattern on MRI.

> ***Note** : Theoretically, any pattern of signal intensity is possible.*

    - In practice, mucoceles are hyperintense on T_2-weighted MRI, and are either hypointense or hyperintense on T_1-weighted sequences. The T_2-weighted sequence will often demonstrate lower signal intensity mucoid concretions within the high signal fluid.

5

Radiology of Bone Diseases (Osteology)

You Should Know

1. The **serum alkaline phosphatase** is not elevated in **multiple myeloma.**
2. Bilateral symmetrical **pseudofractures** or **Looser's lines** indicate → OSTEOMALACIA.
3. Regarding **renal rickets**—
   - Subperiosteal erosions.
   - Azotaemia.
   - Soft tissue calcification.
   - Moth eaten metaphyseal rarefaction.

> ***Note:*** *Depressed blood phosphate level not usually found in renal rickets.*

4. The most prominent finding in **Milk-alkali syndrome** is SOFT TISSUE CALCIFICATION.
5. Vitamin 'D' intoxication in the adult tends to produce → BONE DEMINERALIZATION.
6. **Pseudohypoparathyroidism** is usually accompanied by—
   - Basal ganglia calcification.
   - Increased bone density.
   - Soft tissue calcification.
   - Short stature.

> ***Note:*** *Pseudohypoparathyroidism is usually not accompanied by → PARATHYROID HYPERPLASIA.*

7. **Hypophosphatasia** most closely resembles → RICKETS.

8. Characteristic finding of **hyperparathyroidism** includes—
   - Subperiosteal bone resorption.
   - Periarticular calcification.
   - Cystic bone lesions.
   - Decreased bone density.

> ***Note:*** *PSEUDOFRACTURES is not a characteristic finding of hyperparathyroidism.*

9. Recognised finding of SCURVY includes—
   - Subperiosteal haematoma.
   - Generalized osteoporosis.
   - Transverse radiolucent metaphyseal bands in long bones.
   - Epiphyseal plate fractures.

> ***Note:*** *The finding of metaphyseal cupping is not a part of scurvy.*

10. The findings of a small, dense skull base and flattened acetabular angles indicates → ACHONDROPLASIA.
11. In ELLIS-VAN-CREVALD DISEASE (Chondro-ectodermal dysplasia) the most severe bone changes are found in the **distal extremities.**
12. **Multiple centers of calcification in the epiphysis** are found in **chondrodystrophia calcificans** and occasionally in Achondroplasia and CRETINISM.
13. The finding of **generalized swollen ribs** that show thin cortices and posterior tapering suggests HURLER'S disease or GARGOYLISM.
14. The blood in OSTEOGENESIS IMPERFECTA shows normal calcium (Ca^{++}).
15. The findings of **non-union of the mandibular halves** and of the **zygomatic arches** suggests → CLEIDOCRANIAL DYSOSTOSIS.
16. When bones show a **"Bone within bone"** appearance, this is indicative of → OSTEOPETROSIS.
17. **Coxa vara** in childhood with fragmentation of the femoral neck is probably congenital.

18. The primary anomaly in KLIPPEL-FEIL SYNDROME is **fusion.**
19. A multicystic process without bone reaction in the metaphysis of a long bone of a child is most likely to be → TUBERCULOSIS.
20. **Blastomycosis** or **coccidioidomycosis** may be considered more likely than TUBERCULOSIS of the spine if there is involvement of both bodies and neural arches.
21. Regarding **actinomycosis of the spine**–
    - Involvement of the transverse processes and adjacent ribs.
    - Honeycomb destruction of body with sclerotic lattice work.
    - Large paravertebral abscess.
    - Infrequent vertebral body collapse.

> ***Note:*** *Disc narrowing is not an usual feature of Actinomycosis.*

22. Recognized characteristics of **Brodie's abscess**—
    - Localized radiant abscess in bone.
    - Sclerotic bone.
    - Haematogenous origin of *Staphylococcus* aureus.
    - Chronic course.

> ***Note*** *: Epiphyseal location is not characteristic of Brodie's abscess.*

23. A well-defined **round radiant defect** in the supratrochlear septum of the distal humerus with an included bony body or fragment indicates → OSTEOCHONDRITES DESSICANS.
24. Gradual constriction at the base of the little toe with progressive AUTOAMPUTATION indicates → AINHUM.
25. **Raynaud's syndrome** with classical colour changes, bone atrophy and calcinosis circumscripta is seen with–
    - Raynaud's disease.

- Scleroderma.
- Cryoglobinemia.
- Thromboangiitis obliterans (TAO).

> **Note:** *It is not seen with sickle cell anaemia.*

26. A unilateral painful 2nd rib showing diffuse rarefaction and bone sclerosis with increasing periosteal new bone formation as well as hypertrophy and calcification of the costochondral cartilage suggests probably → TIETZE'S DISEASE.
27. Findings of painful periosteal thickening and cortical hyperostosis with abnormal thinning and premature fusion of the epiphyseal lines of the long bones indicate probably → HYPERVITAMINOSIS–'A'.
28. Leontiasis ossea with its irregular thickening of the skull is probably a form of → FIBROUS DYSPLASIA.
29. A lobulated, expansile, metaphyseal, cystic lesion in an adolescent showing a smudgy appearance of intrinsic calcification with adjacent bone density probably represents–**fibrous dysplasia.**
30. **Skeletal anomalies** such as Kyphoscoliosis, localized growth disturbances and spina bifida as well as cystic lesions in the bony skeleton suggest → NEUROFIBROMATOSIS.
31. Cystic bone lesions with precocious sexual development and irregular pigmentation (Cafe-au-lait) of the back indicate polyostotic fibrous dysplasia (Albright's syndrome).
32. The most common location of **osteogenic sarcoma** is lower femur.
33. The **poor prognosis** in osteogenic sarcoma secondary to Paget's disease is principally due to high vascularity of Paget's disease.
34. An expansile trabeculated lesion in the spine resembling giant cell tumour of the long bones is probably → ANEURYSMAL BONE CYST.
35. Unilateral cortical thickening of long bones mainly on one side of the bones with occasionally

small bone deposits in soft tissues near joints point to → MELORHEOSTOSIS.

36. **Maffucci's syndrome** includes haemangiomatosis and Ollier's disease.
37. The lowest incidence of **unicameral bone cyst** is seen in **radius.**
38. A benign tumour that shows no active growth is **unicameral cyst.**
39. Second to the prostate as a source of metastatic carcinoma in the male is the → LUNG.
40. About **70% of giant cell tumours** occur in the region of the **knee.**
41. The most common carpal fracture is that of the SCAPHOID, the 2nd most common is that of the **triquetrum.**
42. Epiphyseal displacement in childhood are really fractures through the transitional zone of **primary ossification.**
43. X-ray examination in **"pulled elbow"** usually shows no osseous abnormality.
44. The combination of oblique fracture of the proximal ulna and dislocation of the radial head is called MONTEGGIA FRACTURE DISLOCATION.
45. A frequent problem with **fractures of the medial malleolus of the distal tibia** is → interposition of soft tissue.
46. The absence of adequate hepatic **homogentisic acid oxidase** causes → OCHRONOSIS.
47. The average age of onset of **infantile cortical hyperostosis** (Caffey's disease) is → **9 weeks.**
48. Recognized conditions associated with or results in OSTEOMALACIA include—
    - Chronic pancreatitis.
    - Hypophosphatasia.
    - Fanconi's disease.
    - Renal acidosis.

> ***Note:*** *The clinical condition does not result in osteomalacia is → CUSHING'S DISEASE.*

49. **Pyle's disease** and **Gaucher's disease** share a similar finding undertubulation of the distal femora.
50. The finding suggests infantile **cortical hyperostosis** rather than hypervitaminosis 'A' is MANDIBULAR involvement.
51. The injurious agent in **Pseudogout** is calcium pyrophosphate.
52. The hard little knobs in the fingers called HEBERDEN'S NODES are → **Marginal osteophytes**.
53. **Luschka joints** are found in the **cervical spine**.
54. Both knee joints show narrowing, subarticular cystic defects and deep, wide intercondylar fossae indicating probably HEMOPHILIA.
55. The finding favours GOUT rather than RHEUMATOID ARTHRITIS is → **Para-articular bone erosions.**
56. Definite widening of the joints of the hands and spine indicate probable → ACROMEGALY.
57. **Pigmented villonodular synovitis** usually show—
    - Intra- and para-articular nodular masses.
    - Joint effusion.
    - Occasional cystic bone cavities typically on both sides of the joint.
    - Insidious onset in the 3rd to 5th decades.

> ***Note:*** *Pigmented villonodular synovitis does not usually show calcification within the lesions.*

58. GOUT is probable if the **uric acid** level in mg/100 cc of serum is greater than 7.
59. The **blood calcium** (Ca^{++}) level may be elevated in **multiple myeloma**.
60. The **blood phosphate** (PO_4^-) level is usually elevated in **hypoparathyroidism**.
61. The **normal serum phosphorus level for an infant** (under one year of age) is 4 to 6 mg/100 cc.

62. **Normal adult blood serum calcium level** is 8.5 to 10.5 mg/100 cc.
63. Diagnostic findings of SARCOIDOSIS include–
    - Involvement of the distal ends of the proximal and middle phalanges of the hands.
    - Prominent reticulated or lattice-like trabecular pattern of involved bones.
    - Round cysts-like lesions.
    - Occasional prominent destruction.

> ***Note:*** *The finding marks SARCOIDOSIS a less likely diagnosis is → PERIOSTEAL PROLIFERATION.*

64. The most frequent site of **osteochondritis dessicans** is the → MEDIAL FEMORAL CONDYLE.
65. The most prominent effect of **hypogonadism** is → Delayed fusion of the epiphyses.
66. The most prominent bone finding in **Cushing's disease** is → OSTEOPOROSIS.
67. The RADIANT EPIPHYSEAL LINE is generally narrowed rather than widened in → **Hypopituitarism.**
68. Fracture and dorsal dislocation at the proximal end of the 1st metacarpal demands traction and is called **Bennett's fracture dislocation**.
69. **Pellegrini-Stieda's disease** at the medial collateral ligament of the knee is an example of → POST-TRAUMATIC MYOSITIS OSSIFICANS.
70. A rather frequent (25%) and unavoidable complication of transverse fracture of the patella is → ASEPTIC NECROSIS.
71. In posterior dislocation of the femoral head, the femur is usually in prominent → ABDUCTION.
72. Coxa vera may result from—
    - Congenital coxa vara.
    - Legg-Perthes disease.
    - Rickets.
    - Slipped femoral capital epiphysis.

> ***Note:*** *POLIOMYELITIS does not produce coxa vara but coxa valga.*

73. Define osteoporosis, osteomalacia and osteopenia.
    - **Osteoporosis** is a generalized decrease in total bone mass. It is due to insufficient formation or increased resorption of bone matrix.
    - **Osteomalacia** is characterized by poor mineralization of normal, or sometimes increased volumes of osteoid.

> ***Note:*** *In fact, osteomalacia is a qualitative deficiency whereas osteoporosis is a quantitative abnormality.*

- **Osteopenia** ("Poverty of bone") is a general, non-specific term that encompasses both of the above diseases.

> ***Note:*** *This term is used to describe a pathologically decreased quantity of bone when the exact cause of the radiologically decreased bone density is unknown.*

74. Regarding **osteoporosis**—
    - Demographically it is most prevalent in **females**, light hair and eyes, Northern European or Asian ancestry, slender bodily habitus and elderly (senile osteoporosis).
    - **Deficiency states** like poor calcium and/or vitamin D intake, scurvy, malnutrition/anorexia nervosa, excess caffeine and/or alcohol intake, smoking, weightlessness, immobilization/disuse, drugs such as steroids, heparin and phenytoin.
    - Endocrine/systemic cause of osteoporosis.
      a. Endocrine-primary/secondary hyperparathyroidism, Cushing's syndrome oestrogen deficiency (Postmenopausal ladies), hypogonadism (Turner's syndromes, hyperthyroidism and acromegaly).

b. Congenital/genetic-Osteogenesis imperfecta, homocystinuria, mucopolysaccharidoses, sickle cell disease, thalassemia and neuromuscular diseases.

c. Other-Intestinal malabsorption syndrome, neoplastic (e.g. multiple myeloma, metastasis, infiltrative marrow diseases, rheumatoid arthritis, amyloidosis and liver disease.

- Radiographic features useful in diagnosing osteoporosis—
  a. Decrease bony density.
  b. Cortical thinning.
  c. Accentuation of trabecular stress lines due to resporption of secondary trabeculae **(best seen at femoral neck)**.
  d. Prominence of vertebral body end plates.

> ***Note:*** *CT is more sensitive than conventional radiograph for evaluating bone mineral density.*

75. Regarding **single photon absorptiometry** (SPA)—
- SPA was developed in 1960s as a means for quantitative assessment of the bone mineral content at various sites of the **peripheral skeleton.**
- A highly collimated photon beam from a radionuclide (I–125) is used to measure photon attenuation usually at the **distal radius.**
- This technique is most accurate when soft tissue thickness is constant.
- The primary disadvantage of SPA is its inability to provide accurate measurements at sites of variable soft tissue thickness and composition (e.g. spine, hip).

> ***Note:*** *This limitation is overcome by utilizing dual photon absorptiometry (DPA).*

76. Regarding **dual photon absorptiometry (DPA)**—

- DPA utilizes radiation of two distinct energies, one high energy beam and one low energy.
- A high purity high energy activity **Gadolinium–153 source** is utilized providing photons with energies of **44 Kev** and **100 Kev.** The low energy beam is attenuated to a greater degree than the high energy beam.
- In both bone and soft tissue the low-energy beam (44 Kev) is attenuated more than the high energy beam (100 Kev), but to a much greater extent in bone. Therefore, bony yields a higher contrast at low energies than at high energies.

> ***Note:*** *DPA exploits this difference in contrast; entering these attenuation profile into a mathematical equation allows accurate calculation of the bone mineral density of the spine and hip.*

77. Regarding **dual X-ray absorptiometry** (DEXA)—
    - It utilizes the same physical principles as DPA, except that the radionuclide source is replaced with an X-ray tube.
    - Two distinct energy **X-ray beams** are used (usually **70 KVP** and **140 KVP**) and the similar calculation as done in DPA are applied.

> ***Note:*** *DEXA is considered as the state of the art examination for the diagnosis and follow-up of osteoporosis.*

78. Advantages of DEXA over DPA include—
    - Shortened examination time due to greater photon flux of the X-ray tube (lumbar spine evaluation takes 5 to 10 minutes as compared to 20 to 45 minutes for DPA).
    - Better anatomic resolution.
    - Greater accuracy and precision.
    - Comparatively cheaper.
79. Skeletons that are routinely assessed on a DEXA scan include—

- The lumbar spine, from L1 or L2 and the proximal femur (regions of interest in the femoral neck, trochanteric region, and Ward's triangle).

> ***Note:*** *"**Ward's triangle**" is a site at the proximal femur where bone mineral loss is thought to occur first.*

80. A large **osteophytes and sclerotic changes** in a patient with lumbar degenerative disease affect bone densitometry assessment by providing erroneous elevation of the BMD. This can result in the BMD of an osteoporotic patient appearing falsely normal.

> ***Note:*** *This problem is overcome by newer DEXA equipment that allows lateral scanning of the lumbar spine.*

81. Other modalities being evaluated currently for assessing osteoporosis.
    - **Ultrasound scanners** are available for measuring the patella or calcaneus for BMD. This US scanning assessment is relatively inexpensive and devoid of any radiation hazard.
    - **MRI scanning** evaluation of BMD assessment is based on the loss of vertebral bone mineral and concomitant increase in fatty marrow occurring in osteoporosis.
82. Enumerate advantages does MRI offer over other imaging modalities for evaluation of the **musculoskeletal system.**
    - Assessment of B.M. abnormalities, MRI can accurately detect subtle derangements in the composition of bone marrow. Any marrow-replacing process (e.g. infection, tumour) is detected as a diffuse or focal loss of the normally hyperintense fatty marrow signal on **T_1-weighted images.**
    - Detection of occult fractures and bone contusions.

- Visualization of tendons, ligaments, and cartilage.
- Staging of musculoskeletal tumours.

83. Describe the **normal appearance of bone marrow** on MRI:

> ***Note:*** *Fatty and haematopoietic marrow differ in MR appearance.*

- The adult skeleton, containing mostly fatty (yellow) marrow, appears uniformly hyperintense on T_1-weighted images like (fat).
- Haematopoietic (red) marrow, containing much less fat than fatty marrow has lower T_1 signal.

> ***Note:*** *Such haematopoietic marrow predominates in children and in the axial skeleton of adults. The proportion of red marrow in adults becomes relatively increased in chronic anaemia (red marrow reconversion).*

- Haematopoietic marrow also may undergo hyperplasia, particularly in smokers, obese women, and high performance athletes, occasionally resulting in a striking appearance of decreased T_1 signal.

6

Radiology of Cardiovascular System

You Should Know

1. Recognised radiologic findings of **paroxysmal tachycardia** include:
   - Nonspecific cardiomegaly of varying degree.
   - Pulmonary congestion.
   - Occasional isolated left atrial enlargement.
   - Rapid and feeble cardiac pulsation.
2. **Complete heart block** is demonstrated radiologically as—
   - Cardiomegaly.
   - Mostly left ventricular enlargement.
   - Right ventricular and left atrial enlargement.
   - Pulmonary vascular engorgement sometimes.
3. **Pompe's disease** is commonly referred to as cardiac glycogenosis and is **Cori's type II**.
4. **Aortopulmonary fenestration** is a communication between the aorta and the pulmonary artery and the defect is in the → **Anterior wall of the ascending aorta.**
5. In the frontal view of an **oesophagogram** of a patient, there is usually no aortic impression. A marked impression suggests:
   - Hypoplasia of the pulmonary artery.
   - Truncus arteriosus (TA).
   - Aortic stenosis (AS).
   - Persistent ductus arteriosus (PDA).
6. The absence of the normal aortic impression in an **oesophagogram** of an older child speeks for–
   - Transposition.

- Marked counter–clockwise rotation.
- Right aortic arch.
- Hypoplasia of the aorta.

7. The combination of **cyanosis and a large right atrium** mandate the diagnoses of—
   - Total anomalous pulmonary venous return and pulmonary stenosis.
   - Ebstein's and Uhl's anomalies.
   - Tricuspid and pulmonary atresia.
   - Transposition and endocardial cushion defects.
8. Recognized **CVS lesions associated with congenital rubella** include:
   - Persistent ductus arteriosus (PDA).
   - Coarctation of the aortic isthmus.
   - Pulmonary stenosis or hypoplasia.
   - Absence of the inferior vena cava.
9. The **arterial supply to the ipsilateral lung with absence of right pulmonary artery** is derived from the—
   - Ascending aorta.
   - Branch of the aortic arch.
   - Bronchial arteries.
   - Ductus arteriosus.
10. **Rib notching** on X-ray is seen in **coarctation of aorta** (COA).
11. **"Scimitar sign"** is seen in partial anomalous pulmonary venous return (PAPVR).
12. **Kerley's 'A' lines** are seen in **left heart failure.**
13. **"Jonsson's sign"** is present in PDA.
14. VSD and PS is a component of **Fallot's tetralogy.**
15. ASD (R to L) and PS is a component of **Trilogy of Fallot**.
16. ASD (L to R) and PS is a component of **Biology of Fallot.**
17. **Tricuspid atresia** is also called as **Wieland's disease.**

18. **Bland-White-Garland syndrome** is anomalous left coronary artery from pulmonary artery.
19. VSD and pulmonary artery hypertension constitute **Eisenmenger's complex**.
20. ASD and pulmonary artery hypertension constitute **Eisenmenger's syndrome**.
21. **Sussman's bulge** is widened persistent ductus at aortic end.
22. Bulging interventricular septum from left ventricular enlargement is called **Bernheim syndrome**.
23. **Albers-Snellen-Taussig syndrom**e is total anomalous pulmonary venous return (Snowman).
24. A systolic murmur of sudden onset in a patient with AMI may be due to → VSD.
25. The most common radiation-induced heart disease following high-dose radiotherapy (RT) to the thorax is → PERICARDITIS.
26. "Silent" AORTIC DISSECTION is more likely due to **cystic medial necrosis**.
27. Most series agree that the mortality due to right heart catheterization is in the order of 0.5%.
28. **Costophrenic septal lines** (Kerley B lines) are visible when the pulmonary capillary pressure reaches **25 mm Hg**.
29. In **mitral stenosis**, the reversal of the preferential blood flow to the normal lower lungs is more likely due to increased arteriolar resistance.
30. The use of the Valsalva maneuver during fluoroscopy is helpful in the study of—
    - Left to right shunts.
    - Mitral valve disease.
    - Pulmonary hypertension.
31. **Pacemaker wire breakage** is located most commonly at the attachment of the electrode to the heart.
32. The **enlargement of the cardiac silhouette in myxoedema** is due to—
    - Myxoedematous infiltration.
    - Pericardial effusion.

33. During angiocardiography, the mitral valve is best visualized in the → **Right anterior oblique view**.
34. **Ossific nodules in the lungs** have been observed in–
    - Left atrial myxoma.
    - Mitral stenosis.
    - Constrictive pericarditis.
35. **Left atrial enlargement** may help differentiate → VSD.
36. **Prominence of aorta** may help differentiate → PDA.
37. **Right aortic arch** opacifying from a right ventriculogram may indicate tetralogy of Fallot.
38. **Traumatic aortic aneurysms** occur more frequently in the isthmus.
39. The most common underlying cause of dissecting aneurysm is **cystic medial necrosis.**
40. Syndromes associated with dissecting aneurysms include–
    - Ehlers-Danlos syndrome.
    - Turner's syndrome.
    - Marfan's syndrome.
41. Pseudocoarctation of the proximal dissecting aorta is due to **congenital kinking**.
42. The most common cause of chronic cor pulmonale is **obstructive emphysema**.
43. Severe fat embolism is associated with radiological findings resembling → **Pulmonary oedema**.
44. Mitral insufficiency is better demonstrated by → **Cine–angiocardiography**.
45. In arteriosclerotic disease of the limbs, the most common sites of occlusion are **superficial femoral and popliteal.**
46. **Cardiac fluoroscopy** offers very accurate findings in the diagnosis of → Aortic valvular disease.

47. Superior vena cava obstruction is most common in **Bronchogenic carcinoma**.
48. During ANGIOCARDIOGRAPHY, accidental injection of contrast into the myocardium is remarkably well tolerated.
49. A prominent and sharply demarcated pulmonary artery segment and a distinct left ventricular contour in an X-ray chest (PA view) strongly suggests **congenital absence of the pericardium**.
50. **Angiographic identification** of the **crista supraventricularis** is very important in the diagnosis of **tetralogy of Fallot.**
51. Demonstration of marked systolic narrowing of the left ventricular cavity by angiocardiography is characteristic of **idiopathic hypertrophic subaortic stenosis** (IHSS).
52. Narrowing of the left ventricular outflow tract irregular anterior mitral leaflet and mitral regurgitation are angiocardiographic signs of → **Endocardial cushion defect**.
53. In **mitral stenosis** (MS), the presence of left atrial wall calcification implies a high incidence of left atrial thrombosis.
54. **Aneurysms** in the muscular portion of the **ventricular septum** are usually due to → **Myocardial infarction.**
55. The most reliable **angiographic sign of malignancy** in tumours of the thyroid gland is irregular vessels outside the gland arising from the ascending cervical artery.
56. Loss of motor function (paraplegia) secondary to intra-aortic injection of contrast is related to perfusion with contrast of **radicular artery** (of Adam Kiewiez).
57. The **"string of beads"** or **"sausage" appearance** of the **renal artery** is due to **medial fibroplasias with aneurysms**.

58. Regarding **aortic dissection**—
    - Traditionally, the investigation to establish diagnosis of aortic dissection is → **Aortography**.

    > ***Note:*** *Aortography is invasive, needs angiographers to perform, time consuming and needs intravascular contrast.*

    - Other less invasive tests used for aortic dissection includes–Dynamic enhanced CT, transoesophageal echocardiography, and MRI scanning.
59. Regarding radiographic manifestations of **pulmonary oedema**—
    - X-ray shows blunting or back of definition of the margins of the lower lobe blood vessels (caused by dependent, perivascular interstitial oedema and equalization of the size of the vessels in the upper and lower portions of the **lungs**.
    - As pulmonary venous pressure continues to increase, the diameter of the upper lobe pulmonary arteries actually surpases the diameter of the lower lobe vessels, producing the classic radiographic picture of redistribution or cephalization of blood flow.

    > ***Note:*** *Cephalization of blood flow is seen in patients with panacinar emphysema associated with a_1 antitrypsin deficiency or patient with multiple or recurrent pulmonary emboli.*

60. Regarding **Kerley's lines**—

    > ***Note:*** *Histologically Kerley's 'B' lines are same as Kerley 'A' and 'C' lines and perhaps more appropriately known as **septal lines**–represented as **thickened interlobular septa**.*

    - **Interlobular septa** are connective tissue **bands** that divide the lung into secondary pulmonary lobules. Branches of the pulmonary veins and lymphetics travel in the **interlobular septa.**

> ***Note:*** *Fluid that collects in the subpleural interstitial space produces thickening of the interlobar tissues, not to be confused with pleural effusion in the interlobar tissues. Fluid that collects in the interlobular septa produces the Kerley's lines.*

- If the fluid fills peripheral interlobular septa on radiographs multiple short, horizontal linear densities that about the pleural space are seen, which are termed **Kerley 'B' lines**.
- If more **central interlobular septa** become fluid-filled and radiologically apparent, it is known as **Kerley 'A' lines**, that accurate lines radiate outward from the hila are seen.
- **Kerley 'C' lines** refer to a cobweb mesh of linear opacities in the middle portion of the lungs.

> ***Note:*** *Do Kerley lines always indicate pulmonary oedema?*
> ***Ans:*** *Not at all.*

61. One of the simplest ways to **measure heart size** is to measure the distance between the right most extent of the right heart border and the left most extent of the left heart border and then measure the width of the chest at its widest point, from the inner margin of the right ribs to the inner margin of the left ribs. This is called **cardiothoracic ratio.**

> ***Note:*** *Between 25 to 50% is considered normal, 50 to 60% is a gray area and greater than 60% is abonormal.*

62. The technical requirement of a chest radiograph for the accurate estimation of **cardiothoracic ratio** includes–
    - If the patient was X-rayed in the upright position.
    - If the projection is posteroanterior.
    - If the standard 6 feet distance in between the X-ray tube and film.

- If the distance is < 6 feet, then cardiac silhouette will be magnified.

> ***Note:*** *Semierect or supine positioning also makes the heart appear larger as does expiration. It is also seen in pectus excavatum.*

- **True cardiac enlargement** includes pericardial effusion, valvular heart disease (mitral/aortic valvular disease) and cardiomyopathy usually due to ischaemia.

63. The **heart chamber gets enlarged** in MS is **left atrium** while in MR is **left atrium** and **left ventricle**.
64. In AS, a **pressure load is imposed on the left ventricle**, leading to hypertrophy rather than enlargement.
65. In AR, a **volume load is imposed on the left ventricle** and the left ventricle dilates.
66. The **best way to detect individual heart chamber enlargement** is either echocardiography, CAT scan and MRI scan.
67. The chest radiographic findings in LVF generally parallel the **mean left atrial pressure**, more conveniently measured as mean pulmonary capillary wedge pressure.

> ***Note:*** *Pressure (MPCWP) upto approximately 15 mm Hg are normal.*

68. Recognized **radiographic findings in pulmonary oedema**—
    - Blurring of the margins of the central pulmonary vessels especially toward the lung bases.
    - The appearance of Kerley lines—
      – **'A' lines** are diagonally oriented markings in the upper lobes.
      – **'B' lines** are short, linear markings perpendicular to the pleural surfaces of the lower lobes.
      – **'C' lines** are polygonal markings, also in the lower lobes; they are the **most common of the Kerley lines**.

- Thickening of the walls of the bronchi, which is apparent when they are seen on-end.
- If elevated pressures persists, the oedema fluid eventually spills into the alveoli.

69. Regarding **imaging options for detecting coronary artery disease.**
    - A significant **coronary artery stenosis** can be identified directly by **arteriography** as a part of cardiac catheterization or indirectly by observing physiologic alterations under stress.
    - Stress usually means exercise on a **treadmill,** with electrocardiography monitoring.
    - In the face of a 70% or greater narrowing of the cross-sectional area of a coronary artery, the relative perfusion of the myocardium supplied by the artery will decrease, and the ischemic myocardium will lose contractility.
70. Regarding **thallium and technetium nuclear scans** for **myocardial ischemia.**

> ***Note:*** *The decrease in perfusion of the ischaemic region, relative to the remainder of the myocardium is the basis for the radiotracer studies of myocardial ischemia.*

- **Thallium 201** is an analog of potassium and technetium 99 m sestamibi behaves similarly are used for such purpose.

> ***Note:*** *The infarct area fails to take up the radio pharmaceuticals.*

71. Regarding the **imaging studies of pericardial effusion.**
    - Very rarely pericardial effusion can be identified on lateral chest X-ray as a vertically oriented opaque stripe between the anterior heart border with its relatively less opaque epicardial fat and the pericardial fat, which is located superficial to the pericardium. This is referred to as "OREO COOKIE" sign and

is accentuated with the patient in the supine position.

- **Echocardiography** provides an inexpensive, convenient and reliable means of detecting pericardial effusion. It can also provide clues to the presence of cardiac tamponade.
- Further evaluation requires CAT scan or MRI scan to be done. Both scanning systems give better overview of pericardium, looking into the entire mediastinum and identifying co-existing pleural disease.

7

Radiology of Chest Including Lungs

You Should Know

1. The **tracheal bifurcation** is best visualized on left anterior oblique standard view of the chest.
2. The right RETROCARDIAC SPACE is best seen on **right anterior oblique view**.
3. The **right lung** is seen to best advantage on the right anterior oblique view.
4. The carinal angle between the right and left bronchi in the adult is approximately 60° degree.
5. In the adult, the normal **retrotracheal space** equals 0.60 of the diameter of C4.
6. The characteristic of **bronchopulmonary sequestration is** that it has an aortic blood supply.
7. The presence of a cavitary lesion with a "FUNGUS BALL" or MYCETOMA suggests → **Aspergillosis**.
8. Disseminated small nodules with calcification suggests → **Histoplasmosis**.
9. Persistent thin walled cavities suggest → **Coccidioidomycosis**.
10. **"Egg-shell" calcifications** in the hilar nodes suggest SILICOSIS.
11. Scattered infiltrates and pleural thickening or calcification suggest → ASBESTOSIS.
12. Diffuse granularity and hilar enlargements suggest → **Berylliosis**.
13. The **middle lobe** contains the lateral and medial segments.

14. Companion shadows of soft tissue density are frequently seen adjacent to the → **Upper two ribs.**
15. Pleural effusion without evident **lung infiltration is most often due to** → Tuberculosis.
16. Radiation pneumonitis following therapy may be distinguished, inpart, from other pathologic conditions by location.
17. **Stage III silicosis** is manifested by nodules over 3 mm with coalescence.
18. The best method of demonstrating small amounts of pleural fluid is to obtain a film in deep inspiration is **decubitus frontal position.**
19. LYMPHOGENOUS METASTASES in the lung is usually first manifested by parenchymal stranding and hilar enlargement.
20. Patients with **Cushing's disease** may show widening of the mediastinum in the chest.
21. Rib fractures in patients with Cushing's disease characteristically show abundant callus.
22. The sign of greatest value in the diagnosis of **pulmonary emphysema** is change in caliber of the arteries.
23. The commonest site for a foreign body in the tracheobronchial tree is **right lower lobe.**
24. Pseudodiverticulosis or glandular filling on a bronchogram is found in **chronic bronchitis.**
25. The commonest cause of BRONCHOLITHIASIS is → **Tuberculosis.**
26. Formation of a PNEUMATOCOELE suggests **staphylococcal** aetiology of pneumonia.
27. A lung haematoma following trauma may presents as a **cyst.**
28. **Inversion of the left hemidiaphragm and paradoxical movement** may be due to **pleural fluid.**
29. **Rib fractures** are most common in **elderly** age group.
30. The **lordotic view** is valuable in confirming the presence of a lesion in the lung apex and also in the lingular segment.

31. The **expiratory film** is valuable in detecting a **small pneumothorax** because intrapulmonary pressure is diminished.
32. A radiopacity involving the extreme apex of the lung is almost invariably situated in **apical segment**.
33. A **radiopacity in the lateral costophrenic angle** usually lies in the lateral or anterior basal segment.
34. The **silhouette sign** in the chest is based on the premise that an intrathoracic radiopacity will obliterate the border of the heart, aorta, or diaphragm if it is anatomically in contact.
35. An opacity that obliterates the left border of the aortic knob lies in apical posterior segment of the upper lobe.
36. On the **left lateral projection**, the left diaphragm can be distinguished from the right because the anterior border is obliterated.
37. The primary importance of the **air bronchogram** is to localize an intrathoracic lesion as being intrapulmonary.
38. The most direct and **reliable roentgen sign of lobar collapse** is displacement of the interlobar septum.
39. The "HILUM OVERLAY" **sign of Felson** is of help in differentiating mediastinal mass from cardiac enlargement.
40. The "THYMIC WAVE" sign is due to **cardiac motion**.
41. If on the frontal projection, the upper border of a superior mediastinal lesion is visible above the clavicles, the **"cervicothoracic" sign of Felson** indicates that the lesion is intrathoracic.
42. A posterior lobulation of the left diaphragm should be further studied most pertinently with **excretory urography**.
43. ROENTGEN KYMOGRAPHY utilizes a slit lead screen and requires movement during the exposure of the Film.

44. **Teratomas of the mediastinum** are almost invariably located in the anterior compartment.
45. The commonest lesions in the posterior mediastinum arise from **neurogenic elements**.
46. **Laceration of the diaphragm following trauma** is most common on the **left side**.
47. An **elevated right hemidiaphragm** following abdominal trauma should suggests rupture of the diaphragm.
48. **Extramedullary haemopoiesis** is usually manifested in the chest by posterior paravertebral mass.
49. Roentgenographically, **chickenpox pneumonia** is characterized by → NODULAR INFILTRATE.
50. The roentgenogram of patients with **pulmonary alveolar proteinosis** may resemble pulmonary oedema pattern.
51. Roentgenologically, **desquamatic interstitial pneumonia** presents most often as → BASILAR INFILTRATE.
52. **Post-traumatic fat embolism** to the lung most often resembles → Pulmonary oedema pattern.
53. Resorption of the superior borders of the posterior aspects of the upper ribs is most characteristic of **collagen disease**.
54. **Kerley B-lines** occur most frequently at the basal region.
55. **Kerley 'B' lines represent** thickened interlobular septa.
56. **Pulmonary microlithiasis** is typified by minute calcific deposits and few symptoms.
57. The **transverse thoracis muscle** is most apt. to be confused with a inferior retrosternal mass.
58. **Childhood tuberculosis** is most often characterized by infiltrate and nodal enlargement.
59. Haemoptysis, haematuria, pulmonary infiltrates and nephritis suggest → **Goodpasture's syndrome**.

60. The most frequent finding following a fracture of the trachea or bronchus is → INTERSTITIAL AIR.
61. Following trauma to the chest an increasing HAEMOTHORAX suggests that the bleeding source is NOT from the lung.
62. Dilatation of the upper lobe (lung) veins is a reliable sign of **cardiac decompensation**.
63. Radiologically RETROPLEURAL HAEMATOMAS are frequently found following → **Sympathectomy**.
64. The presence of **rheumatoid joint disease** in patients with **silicosis** (CAPLAN'S SYNDROME) is manifested by **lung nodules**.
65. The presence of sinusitis with bone destruction and **pulmonary nodules** suggests → WEGENER'S NECROTIZING GRANULOMATOSIS.
66. **Pseudobronchiectasis** or **reversible bronchiectasis** may occur following → LOBAR PNEUMONIA.
67. **Pulmonary melioiodosis** resembles roentgenologically → T.B.
68. Chronic obstructive PSEUDOEMPHYSEMA, SWYER–JAMES MACLEOD syndrome is manifested by **unilateral hyperlucent lung**.
69. The most debilitating feature of **progressive sarcoid** in the lung is → FIBROSIS.
70. The 5 clinical manifestations of rheumatoid lung includes—
    - Chronic pneumonia.
    - Diffuse fibrosis.
    - Nodules.
    - Caplan's syndrome.
    - Pleural effusion.

> ***Note:*** *The commonest clinical manifestations is diffuse fibrosis in rheumatoid lung.*

71. The commonest radiological appearance of a **pulmonary hamartoma** is → COIN LESION.
72. The typical radiological lesion of **Paragonimiasis** is → **Rib erosion**.

73. The **nodular pattern** often seen in the lungs following renal transplantation is thought to be due to → CMV (Cytomegalovirus).
74. The most reliable sign of **diaphragmatic paralysis** is → **Mediastinal shift**.
75. **Heroin overdose** may present with the **pulmonary oedema**.
76. **Farmer's lung** usually manifests roentgenographically as → **Diffuse nodularity**.
77. **Kartagener's triad** consists of paranasal sinusitis, bonchiectasis and situs inversus.
78. Hilar and mediastinal node enlargement in **Hodgkin's disease** is most often **bilateral** and **asymmetrical**.
79. Pleural involvement in sarcoid is very rare.
80. Most solitary tumours of the lung are not perceptible until they exceed → **6 mm**.
81. **Middle lobe collapse** may be demonstrated to best advantage on the **lordotic projection**.
82. The most important considerations when **evaluating a patient who has chest injuries** include the **ABCs**–airway, breathing and circulation, are the 1st priority in all trauma cases.
83. Regarding the ABCDE approach to guide the Radiologic search for thoracic injuries–
    - **Air**–Extrapulmonary (Pneumothorax, pneumomediastinum, pneumopericardium, pneumoperitoneum, subcutaneous emphysema).
    - **Aorta**–Traumatic rupture of aorta.
    - **Bones**–Thoracic spine fractures, other less important fractures are ribs, scapula, sternum.
    - Contusions and lung lacerations.
    - Catheter (vascular) and tube placement.
    - Diaphragm – Rupture.
    - Effusions – Hemothorax.

> ***Note:*** *The radiographic search for these injuries should be undertaken only after the patient has been clinically assessed and stabilized. Since most trauma victims are X-rayed while supine or semi-recumbent, abnormalities such as pneumothorax and hemothorax may hook different than they would on an erect chest X-ray.*

84. The best way to diagnose a **pneumothorax in a trauma victim** is a CAT scan of thorax and upper abdomen.
85. If the classic findings of pneumothorax are not present on a supine chest radiograph the other clues might be helpful in diagnosing a pneumothorax includes—
    - The **deep sulcus sign:** Abnormal deepening of the costophrenic angle on the affected side.
    - The **double diaphragm sign:** The anterior prosterior interfaces of the diaphragm with air (anteriorly with the pneumothorax, posteriorly with the lung) can be seen creating the impression of two diaphragms on the affected side.
    - Visualization of pericardial fat.
    - Basilar hyperlucency.
86. When the X-ray chest suggests the possibility of **aortic injury** and the patient is haemodynamically unstable then the direct inspection of the aorta in the operating room is indicated.

    If there is an apparent extrathoracic source of bleeding, particularly in the abdomen, the patient can undergo a laparotomy, and a transoesophageal US examination of the aorta (**Transoesophageal echocardiography** or TEE) can be performed simultaneously. This test is **very sensitive and specific** for diagnosing TRAUMATIC AORTIC RUPTURE and can be done with portable equipment in OT itself.
87. If the chest radiograph suggests aortic injury, but the patient is haemodynamically stable, evaluation can be done by using either of the 3 test like CAT scan, TEE and aortography.

> ***Note:*** *AORTOGRAM is regarded as the gold standard test for diagnosing* ***aortic rupture****.*

- Patients who have grossly abnormal mediastinal or aortic silhouttes often go directly to aortography because of the perceived high probability of aortic rupture.

> **Note:** *The main disadvantage of aortography is its invasiveness, expensiveness and time consuming.*

88. The dynamic contrast-enhanced helical CAT scan of the chest can reliably detect or exclude aortic injury and should be done routinely in all patients.

> **Note: Helical CAT scan** *can be done in < 10 minutes, image the entire thoracic aorta and can demonstrate other injuries in the chest and abdomen.*

89. **"Aortic nipple"** is a focal bulge in the lateral aspect of the aortic knob produced by the left superior intercostals vein.

> **Note:** *On plain X-ray chest (PA view), the aortic nipple may be mistaken for mediastinal adenopathy, while on CAT scan of chest, the left superior intercostals vein may be mistaken for aortic dissection.*

90. Conditions mimicing pneumonia on chest radiograph.

- Lung cancer may mimic pneumonia by producing a postobstructive pneumonia or a "drowned" lobe or lung.
- When a neoplasm occludes a bronchus, sloughed cells, secretions, and transuded fluid accumulate distal to the site of obstruction, producing a radiographic opacity called a **postobstructive pneumonia**.
- Infection is usually absent and if the obstruction ensues slowly the volume of the affected lobe or segment may be maintained or may increase.
- Bronchoalveolar lung C_A (a type of adenocarcinoma lung).
- Pulmonary lymphoma.
- Aspiration.

- Haemorrhage.
- Pulmonary oedema (cardiogenic or non-cardiogenic).
- Sarcoidosis.
- Lipoid pneumonia.
- Alveolar proteinosis.

91. **X-ray appearance of *Pneumocystis carinii* pneumonia (PCP) in patients with HIV infection (AIDS)**

> **Note:** *PCP is the most common cause of morbidity and mortality in patient who have AIDS.*

- Typically PCP causes bilateral symmetric perihilar opacities, and death resulted or the pneumonia cleared completely.

> **Note:** *Although bilateral symmetric opacities are the most common X-ray findings in HIV–positive patient with PCP, an impressive array of varied radiographic abnormalities have been demonstrated:*

- Focal air space opacities.
- Hilar and/or mediastinal lymphadenopathy (sometimes calcified).
- Pleural effusion.
- Cavities.
- Bilateral upper lobe cysts.

92. In **HIV positive patients with T.B. cavitation** is less commonly seen because cavitation requires the presence of relatively intact CMI. HIV positive patient whose **CD4 counts are above 200 cmm may produce cavitation**, whereas patients whose CD4 counts are below 200 cmm are much less likely to develop cavitation.

8

Radiology of Gastrointestinal System

You Should Know

1. Radiologically **pleural effusion** is demonstrable in—
   - Pancreatitis.
   - Subhepatic abscess.
   - Subphrenic abscess.
   - Ovarian fibroma.

   > ***Note:*** *It is not commonly associated with splenic infarct.*

2. The minimum volume of free intraperitoneal gas that can be visualized roentgenographicaly is **1 cc**.
3. **Abnormalities within the lesser sac** are recognized by a large left sided soft tissue density with an oblique lower border.
4. **Blunt abdominal trauma** affects the GIT most commonly at the 2nd portion of the duodenum.
5. By employing both the hepatic angle and the flank strike signs, diagnostic accuracy of **ascites** should approach **97%**.
6. The **incidence of positive diagnosis of mechanical small bowel obstruction** on the basis of plain abdominal film is **55%**.
7. The average transit time in the normal small bowel is **85 minutes**.
8. The commonest cause of **calcified splenic cysts** is parasitic infestations.
9. Markedly distended **jejunum differs from** similarly distended **ileum** in that thin valvulae

persist in the jejunum but often disappear in the ileum.

10. **Splenoportography** done in the presence of portal hypertension reveals that the collateral filling is obtained in all cases.
11. **Portal venography** via injection of the coeliac or splenic anteries is useful in determining:
    - Existence of collateral channels in portal hypertension.
    - Patency of a portocaval shunt.
    - Patency of a portal vein.
12. **Portal venography via arterial route** is superior to splenoportography because it can be performed—
    - In the presence of ascites.
    - In the absence of spleen.
    - In the presence of small spleen.
    - In the presence of an infected spleen.
13. **Hepatic** and/or **splenic angiography** in the Budd-Chiari syndrome demonstrates:
    - Intense and prolonged hepatogram.
    - Prolonged opacification of the spleen.
14. **Metastases to the liver** show increased vascularity commonly from the malignant islet cell tumour of the pancreas (Primary site).
15. **Angiographically,** hepatomas reveals—
    - Have large feeding arteries.
    - Commonly display tumour vessels.
16. **Angiographically,** cavernous haemangiomas—
    - Usually do not have a major increase in the number of arterial vessels.
    - Cause crowding of major intrahepatic vessels.
17. When carefully performed, **oral cholecystography** has a diagnostic accuracy of **95%**.
18. The incidence of **opaque biliary calculi** is about **20%**.
19. **Emphysematous cholecystitis** is found mainly in patients with poorly controlled diabetes mellitus.

20. **Oral cholecystography** is unlikely to be successful in patient with serum bilirubin above **1.0 mg%**.
21. **Neoplasm of the gallbladder** usually are discovered in a non-functioning gallbladder.
22. The commonest **site of impaction of the stone in gallstone ileus** is at the **distal ileum**.
23. **Opacification of the gallbladder** during I.V. cholangiography **does not occur** in acute cholecystitis.
24. The **presence of opaque gallstones in children** or young adults is usually associated with HAEMOLYTIC ANAEMIAS.
25. The optimal time interval between ingestion of oral cholecystographic pills and filming is 10 hours.
26. The **"Coffee bean" sign** indicates–strangulation of an incompletely obstructed loop of small bowel.
27. The **"pseudotumour of Frimann-Dahl"** is encountered in strangulation of a completely obstructed loop of small bowel.
28. **Traumatic rupture of the diaphragm** occurs most frequently at the posterior portion of the left hemidiaphragm.
29. **Calculi in the appendix** in combination with acute appendicitis indicate that the appendix most likely is gangrenous and frequently perforated.
30. KILLIAN'S DEHISCENCE is a potential weak spot between the oblique and transverse fibres of the **cricopharyngeus**.
31. **Hypopharyngeal webs** never occur on the posterior wall.
32. **Oesophageal ulcers** occur with gastric or duodenal ulcer, hiatus hernia or in islets of heterotopic gastric mucosa.
33. **Intramural diverticulosis of the oesophagus** may be post-operative hiatus hernia, alkaline oesophagitis and oesophageal stricture.

34. **Dysphagia lusoria** is associated with aberrant right subclavian artery.
35. The **most significant finding in GIT amyloidosis** is motor dysfunction.
36. In "ACHALASIA OF THE OESOPHAGUS" beyond the initial stage normal peristalsis is abolished and disorganized contractions appear.
37. "GRANULOMATOUS GASTRITIS" may simulate scirrhous carcinoma, lues (syphilis) and tuberculosis.
38. **"Prolapse of the mucosa of the stomach"** into the duodenum occurs commonly and is asymptomatic.
39. A SOL (Space occupying lesion) in the small bowel, that can be obliterated by compression is characterized by a VARIX.
40. The "TOBACCO-POUCH" stomach is due to **lye ingestion**.
41. The **"Zollinger-Ellison syndrome"** should be strongly suspected when the patient has persistent haematemesis.
42. The **"afferent loop syndrome"** refers to preferential emptying of the gastric remnant into the proximal loop of a gastrojejunostomy leading to stasis, vit. B_{12} deficiency and resulting anaemia.
43. The **"Zollinger-Ellison syndrome"** is hypophycemia, fainting and weakness after eating.
44. The **post-gastrectomy dumping syndrome** consists of weakness, sweating, tachycardia associated with a feeling of fullness, cramps, diarrhoea and nausea shortly after eating.
45. **Primary enterolithiasis** is indicative of a Mecket's diverticulum or stenosing disease of the small bowel.
46. The **"Peutz-Jegher syndrome"** consists of oral and skin pigmentation associated with multiple hamartomatous polyps of the small bowel and colon.

47. **Elevated urinary 5-hydroxyindoleacetic acid** levels are found in the CARCINOID SYNDROME.
48. **Multiple polypoid lesions** of the terminal ileum in patient's with colonic polyposis and GARDNER'S syndrome are most likely to be lymphoid hyperplasia.
49. The **roentgen manifestations of disaccharidase deficiency** are rapid transit time, dilatation of loops and dilution of barium on small bowel studies.
50. An exudative inflammation that involves primarily the mucosa, secondarily the submucosae and only occasionally the muscularis is ULCERATIVE COLITIS.
51. The roentgen findings of skip lesions, longitudinal ulcerations, eccentric involvement, pseudodiverticula, stricture formation, pseudopolypi, internal fistulae and sinus tracts are characteristics of **granulomatous colitis**.
52. "SENTINEL POLYPS" are found adjacent to a colonic C_A in as many as 30% of the cases.
53. A **single contrast upper G1 series film** shows following parts of stomach, like– gastroesophageal junction, cardia, fundus, body, antrum, and pylorus.
54. The normal mucosal pattern of the stomach is called as **area gastricae** which is observed on double contrast studies.
55. **On a plain X-ray abdomen**, the structures that may normally contain gas is **stomach** and **colon**.
56. A **single/double contrast barium enema film** shows the following parts of colon like–Ileocaecal valve, caecum, appendix, ascending colon, transverse colon, descending colon, sigmoid colon and rectum.
57. **Oblique view of the thoracic oesophagus** from a single contrast barium swallow shows normal areas of indentation from adjacent

structures includes–Aortic knob, left main stream bronchus, left atrium, diaphragmatic hiatus.

58. The parts of the biliary tree and pancreatic ducts that may be seen on an ERCP.

Biliary tree	*Pancreatic duct*
• Right and left hepatic ducts	• Head
• Common hepatic duct	• Body
• Cystic duct	• Tail
• Gallbladder	
• Common bile duct	

59. **Abdominal organs** routinely seen on an **abdominal U.S.** (Ultrasound).
    - Liver.
    - Gallbladder.
    - Spleen.
    - Pancreas.
    - Kidneys.
60. **Ultrasound** (US) demonstrate less than 3 mm the normal gallbladder wall thickness.
61. Enumerate radiologic studies that can be used to image the oesophagus.
    - Barium oesophagogram.
    - CAT/MRI scan.
    - Endoscopic ultrasound.
62. Regarding **Schatzki's ring**—
    - It is named for Richard Schatzki, German born American Radiologist (1901-1992).
    - It is a thin, ring-like constriction of the distal oesophagus measuring 2 to 5 mm in height.
    - The **ring** may vary in the degree of its constriction, producing the classic symptoms of dysphagia for solid to a greater degree than liquids.

> ***Note:*** *Symptoms are particularly common when the diameter at the ring is less than 13 mm.*

- The **oesophagogram view** best demonstrates a Schatzki's ring is the distal oesophagus obtained with the patient prone and is a slight right anterior oblique position.

63. The tumour may occur in the oesophagus of AIDS patients is **Kaposi's sarcoma**. The X-ray appearance is that of multiple polypoid lesions or submucosal masses, which may ulcerate producing a **target appearance**.
64. Regarding the **causes of GIT haemorrhage** in AIDS—
    - AIDS is associated with **infection** and neoplasm of the GIT, which can occasionally result in haemorrhage.
    - The **neoplastic causes of GI haemorrhage** in AIDS include Kaposi's sarcoma and lymphoma.
    - The primary infectious aetiology is CMV colitis.

> ***Note:*** *In most cases, arteriography enables localization of the bleeding site and facilitates transcatheter treatment with embolic agents or vasoconstrictive drugs.*

65. For **scintigraphic examination** Tc-99m labeled red cells and Tc-sulphur colloid are available for lower GIT bleeding.

> ***Note: Scintigraphy*** *is more sensitive for detecting GI hemorrhage than* ***arteriography*** *because bleeding rates as low as* ***0.1 ml/minutes*** *can be detected, while arteriography usually requires a bleeding rate of 0.5 to 1.0 ml/minutes for detection.*

66. The **Tc-99m labelled red cells scan** is superior to sulphur colloid scan for detecting GIT bleeding.
67. The **radiologic findings in gastritis** on an upper GI series include–Erosions, thickened folds, nodules, and polyps.

> ***Note:*** *Each of these findings may be found alone or in combination.*

68. The most common location for **gastric erosions** is the antrum.
69. Recognised **radiologic signs of a benign gastric ulcer** includes—
    - **Projection of the ulcer crater** beyond the expected location of the gastric wall.
    - **Hampton's line:** A thin, sharply demarcated line with parallel, straight margins at the base of the ulcer crater.
    - **Ulcer collar:** A lucent ring that separates the ulcer crater from the gastric mucosa.
    - **Ulcer mound**, which is caused by mucosal oedema.
70. Recognized **radiologic sign of a malignant gastric ulcer** includes—
    - **Gastric folds** do not reach the edge of the ulcer crater.
    - **Gastric folds** are irregular, amputated, or clubbed.
    - **Ulcer crater** does not project beyond the expected location of the gastric wall.
    - **Carman's meniscus sign** and the **Kirkland complex**.
      - The **Carman's meniscus** refers to a finding described on a single contrast barium examination, where compression of the edges of a malignant ulcer causes the walls of the ulcer to touch and trap barium. The trapped barium is located in the ulcer bed, which has a meniscoid appearance–the inner margin is concave toward the lumen.
    - The **Kirkland complex** refers to the heaped margins of the ulcer, which touch. This projects as a lucent rim around the ulcer on upper GI studies where the anterior abdominal wall is compressed by the radiologist.
71. The most common cell type in gastric cancer is ADENOCARCINOMA in 95% of all gastric neoplasms.

72. Patients with **pernicious anaemia** are at increased risk of developing **gastric cancer**.
73. Radiologic findings in **duodenitis** includes thickening of the duodenal folds is the most sensitive but least specific sign. The folds are generally > 5 mm thick. Other signs include mucosal nodularity, erosions and deformity of the folds.
74. The best imaging test to diagnose the complications of appendicitis is a **contrast-enhanced CT scan**.
75. The best imaging test for **diverticulitis** is CAT scan.
76. Recognized **plain film** and **CT findings** in **ischemic colitis**—
    - Thickening of the colonic wall, with luminal narrowing and transverse ridging.
    - **"Thumb printing"** of the bowel wall, due to oedema.
    - Fixed, rigid, tubular, ahaustral bowel loops.
    - **Pneumatosis** (gas in the bowel wall).
    - Free gas in the peritoneal cavity (uncommon) or in the mesenteric veins and portal vein.

> ***Note:*** *Gas in the mesenteric veins and portal vein are especially ominous and indicate progression of ischemia to infarction.*

77. The early findings of **Crohn's disease** on a barium enema is superficial mucosal ulcers, which look like small bull's eyes (aphthous ulcers).
78. An early finding of **ulcerative colitis** on a barium enema includes a granular pattern a bowel mucosa.
79. Recognised **common signs of small bowel obstruction on plain X-ray**
    - Multiple air fluid levels.
    - Absence of colonic distention.
    - A "stepladder" appearance of small bowel loops/air fluid levels with unequal heights in loops of small bowel.

- **"String of pearls"** which refers to a small amount of residual air in the fluid-filled small bowel loops.

80. CAT scan is the imaging test of choice in patients with **suspected bowel obstruction**.
81. The most common cause of small bowel obstruction is **adhesions**.
82. Recognized CT findings in closed-loop obstruction includes—
    - A 'U' shaped bowel loop.
    - A **"beak" sign** is also found at both narrowed ends of the bowel loop.
    - The mesentery may be seen converging toward the root of the obstruction (the **"whorl" sign**).
83. The best imaging test for staging **pancreatitis** is contrast-enhanced CAT scan.
84. Recognized **complications of pancreatitis** that can be identified on CT includes haemorrhage, pseudocyst formation, pseudoaneurysm formation and development of pancreatic abscess or necrosis.
85. The most common tumour of **pancreas** is **adenocarcinoma**.
86. The **best non-invasive test for staging pancreatic cancer** is contrast-enhanced CT scan.
87. A tumour of the pancreatic head produces **"double duct" signs** which can be seen on CT, US and ERCP.
88. The **"Chain-of-lakes"** appearance of the pancreatic duct as seen on an ERCP in patients with chronic pancreatitis.

> **Note:** *Alternating areas of narrowing and dilatation give this appearance. Also, filling defects such as stones and sludge can be identified.*

89. Most common islet cell tumour is INSULINOMAS.

> **Note:** *Insulinomas are benign tumour rest other islet cell tumours are malignant in nature.*

90. The most common benign tumour of liver is **haemangioma.**

> ***Note:*** *A haemangioma is most commonly found in the posterior segment of the right hepatic lobe. These are more commonly seen in women.*

91. On contrast-enhanced CT or MRI, **haemangioma** usually have a very specific appearance. Initial images show peripheral discontinuous nodular contrast enhancement. Delayed images show more uniform contrast enhancement of the lesion. This appearance is so characteristic that usually no additional work-up is required on T_2-weighted MR images, they are very bright.
92. In **nuclear medicine study**, a radiolabelled RBC scan is diagnostic of HAEMANGIOMA (Tc-99 m tagged RBC).
93. **Tumours commonly metastasize to liver** includes GIT tumours especially colorectal cancer, breast CA and lung CA.

> ***Note:*** *Virtually any tumour may metastasize to the liver.*

94. The **imaging test** most often used to look for **liver metastases** is a contrast-enhanced CT scan and where iodinated contrast is contra-indicated MRI is the 1st choice but expensive than CT scan.
95. The most common benign intramural gastric tumour is → LEIOMYOMA.
96. Recognized **radiologic appearances of gastric cancer on an upper GI series** includes:
    - **Polypoid mass** with or without ulceration and with or without nodularity.
    - **Flat superficial spreading cancer**, sometimes with very shallow ulcerations.
    - Scirrhous submucosally infiltrating carcinomas **(leather bottle stomach)**.
97. **Enumerate primary tumours** most commonly **metastasize to the stomach.**
    - Melanoma.
    - Breast cancer.

- Kaposi's sarcoma.
- Pancreatic cancer.
- Colonic cancer.

98. The most common causes of **haematogenous metastases to the small bowel** are melanoma and bronchogenic CA.
99. The **best test for gallstone** is ultrasound (US) which is non-invasive and very accurate.

> ***Note:*** *On plain X-ray, only 20% of gallstones are visible.*

100. A nuclear medicine test called an HIDA scan, is very accurate in establishing or excluding the diagnosis of **acute cholecystitis**.

> ***Note: Ultrasound*** *shows* ***anatomy better****, while* ***HIDA scan*** *gives the ideas of* ***physiology*** *better.*

101. **Ultrasound** is the best initial test to visualize **dilated bile ducts**.
102. **Patients with IBD** (inflammatory bowel disease) Crohn's disease are at increased risk of developing → **Gallstones** and **urinary tract stones**.
103. About **80%** of **urinary calculi** are visible on plain films or X-ray.
104. The most sensitive imaging test for **abdominal calcification** is CAT scan.
105. A focal area of **"Sun burst"** calcification is seen in the liver on plain X-ray film or CT scan is HAEMANGIOMA.
106. About radiographic examination useful in evaluating IBD–
    - **Barium enema**–used cautiously in active disease, contraindicated with toxic megacolon – for evaluating the extent of colonic disease and complications such as **cancer**.
    - Small bowel follow-through–for evaluating the small bowel, especially the **ileum**.
    - CT–for detecting complications like **fistula** and **abscess formation**.
    - ERCP–for evaluating suspected **sclerosing cholangitis**.

9

Radiology of Genitourinary System

You Should Know

1. Non–visualization of kidney on excretory urography in a patient suspected of having a RENAL CELL CARCINOMA should suggest → RENAL VEIN INVOLVEMENT.
2. Psammomatous-like calcification seen in the suprapubic region of a male pelvis may be seen in the presence of → Bladder neoplasm.
3. The accuracy of nephrotomography is lowest when used to diagnose 1° aldosteronism.
4. During excretory urography, the radiologic findings seen in acute renal vein thrombosis include:
   - Compression of renal pelvis.
   - Enlargement of renal shadow.
   - Diminished function.
   - Beading of ureter.
5. The 1st pyelographic change in RENAL TUBERCULOSIS is in the "Renal pyramid".
6. Xanthogranulomatous pyelonephritis is characterized by—
   - Non-function of kidney.
   - Pyelocalyceal changes suggestive of long-term chronic pyelonephritis.
   - Nephrectomy is the usual form of treatment.
   - Varying degrees of obstructive changes.
7. In chain cysto-urethrography, stress incontinence is indicated by a posterior urethrovesical angel of 125°.
8. Vesico-sigmoidal fistulas are most frequently caused by → DIVERTICULITIS.

9. During acute renal colic, peripelvic extravasation of contrast may be seen during pyelography. This occurs due to egress at the calyceal fornix.
10. The earliest change of chronic pyelonephritis may be increased forniceal angle.
11. Multiple ureteral strictures are almost diagnostic of TUBERCULOSIS.
12. In acute renal obstruction, the nephrogram seen on delayed films during pyelography is due to contrast material in tubules and tubular cells.
13. The majority of "ADRENAL CALCIFICATIONS" are a result of clinically insignificant disease.
14. CYSTITIS EMPHYSEMATOSA (Air within the wall) is usually seen in diabetes mellitus.
15. Calcification of renal cortex might be helpful to distinguish renal brucellosis from renal T.B.
16. Finding a "BEADED APPEARANCE" of the VAS DEFERENS during a vesiculogram indicates → TUBERCULOSIS.
17. Putty kidney is associated with tuberculosis.
18. EXSTROPHY OF URINARY BLADDER is always associated with separation of the symphysis pubis.
19. In pyeloureteritis cystica, the multiple small filling defects noted on excretory urograms contain → SEROUS FLUID.
20. In TUBEROUS SCLEROSIS, one may expect to find renal tumours at autopsy in 80% of cases.
21. The association of cerebellar haemangioblastoma with renal cyst is known as → LINDAU'S DISEASE.
22. The "URETERAL JET phenomenon" in the urinary bladder represents normal propulsion of urine in the bladder.
23. The commonest cystic disorder in infants is unilateral renal dysplasia.
24. **Nephrocalcinosis** is associated with—
    - Cystinuria.
    - 1° hyperoxaluria.
    - Glycinuria.
    - Hypervitaminosis 'D'.

25. In renal artery fibromuscular dysplasia, the right renal artery is predominantly involved when disease is unilateral.
26. Distinguishing ANGIOLIPOMA from RENAL CELL CARCINOMA angiographically is possible when typical microaneurysms are seen without arteriovenous shunting.
27. The "CRESCENT SIGN" of DUNBAR is seen in → HYDRONEPHROSIS.
28. The commonest cause of RENAL INFARCT is → Embolus.
29. **Horseshoe kidney** has markedly increased incidence in → GONADAL DYSGENESIS.
30. In **renal angiography of hydronephrosis,** the decrease of the main artery to less than 50% of normal size indicates poor potential function when obstruction is relieved.
31. **Visualization of the gallbladder** following the injection of IVP contrast media represents more commonly seen in cases with renal dysfunction.
32. **Infiltrative carcinoma of the renal pelvis on renal angiography** may reveal—
    - Predominant parenchymal involvement.
    - Encasement of parenchymal vessels.
    - Hypovascular mass.
    - Enlarged pelviureteric vessel.
33. The **"calyceal crescent"** seen on excretory urogram
    - Indicates obstructive uropathy.
    - Is due to distorted collecting tubules.
    - Is associated with elevated intrapelvic pressure.
34. Regarding **tumefactive xanthogranulomatous pyelonephritis**—
    - May closely resemble hypernephroma.
    - May extend into perinephric tissues.
    - Is characterized by lipid-laden foam cells.
    - Reveals conspicuous absence of Michaelis-Gutman bodies.
35. Regarding renal abnormality in **Von Hippel's disease** (Retinal angiomatosis)–

- Renal cysts and benign tumours.
- Hypernephroma.
- Haemangioendothelioma.

36. Regarding **renal sinus lipomatosis**—
    - May be a normal variant.
    - Commonly seen in obese patients.
    - May disappear when individual loses weight.
    - Nephrotomography is the investigation of choice.
37. **Opacification of collecting tubules during IV urography** results from the steeps rise in concentration in the collecting tubules of the well-dehydrated patient.
38. Regarding **contrast media reactions** the most helpful means to reduce death rate is to ensure that resuscitation drugs (Adrenaline, hydrocortisone, aminophylline) and equipment are immediately available.
39. Regarding the HUTCH diverticulum–
    - Is very commonly seen as an acquired diverticulum associated with trabaculated neurogenic bladder.
    - Causes the intramural ureter to become extravesical like a fixed tube allowing free vesicoureteral reflux.
    - Hutch has named his concept of ureterectasis (inert displaced intramural ureter) plus reflux as "Hydro-flux".
40. Regarding **mullerian duct cysts**—
    - May be selectively catheterized through the utricle and demonstrated radiographically.
    - May be so huge as to displace ureter.
41. Regarding **renal artery aneurysms**—
    - About 60% are discernible as calcifications on plane films: 20% are bilateral and 30% are multiple.
    - Small (<1.5 cm in diameter) calcified true aneurysms in a normotensive patient pose no danger and require no treatment.
42. Regarding DUPLEX kidney–
    - Is 1 to 3 cm larger than contralateral normal non-duplex mate.

- Lobar dysmorphism between upper and lower renal segments is apt. to be mistaken as a "mass lesion".
- Reflux is more common from the orifice of the lower-pole ureterovesical junction.
- Obstruction more commonly affects the upper-pole ureter because its orifice is frequently ectopic.

43. Regarding **roentgenologic visualization of the placenta**—
    - Placental calcification is seen in 90% after 36 weeks provided first rate soft tissue technique is applied.
    - Arterial and isotopic placentography are the most dependable techniques.
44. Regarding vaginal stone on a plain X-ray of the abdomen–
    - May be due to calcification around a foreign body.
    - Forms primarily in vagina due to continuous leakage of urine into the vagina via fistula or as result of urinary incontinence.
45. Metastases to kidney are—
    - Twice as common as primary tumours.
    - Frequently bilateral.
46. Angiogrpahic findings in lymphoma include–
    - Vascular displacement of vessels around the mass.
    - Irregular junction of the tumour with the normal kidney.
    - Irregular capillary stain.
    - Malignant neovasculature.
47. **Angiographic parameters indicating renal graft rejection** include—
    - Altered cortico-pyramidal ratio.
    - Renal swelling.
    - Pyramidal swelling.
48. The commonest **urinary calculus** consists of calcium or magnesium phosphate.
49. **Renal tubular acidosis** radiographically presents as diffuse nephrocalcinosis with **staghorn calculi**.

50. Hapatic fibrosis and dilated bile ducts may be associated with **medullary sponge kidney**.
51. **Medullary cystic disease** leads to chronic anemia, azotemia and salt-losing nephropathy in early adulthood and causes Addisonian like-syndrome.
52. **Tramway** (double line) **calcification** is characteristic radiologic finding in bilateral renal cortical necrosis.
53. Small kidneys with diffuse granular cortical calcification are seen in **chronic glomerulonephritis**.
54. **Hypophosphatasia** often develops in RTA (Renal tubular acidosis) leading to **renal rickets** in children and **osteomalacia** in adults.
55. The most basic radiographic study of the urinary tract is IVP or IVU or excretory pyelography.
56. The most common type of renal artery dysplasia is medial fibroplasia or fibromuscular dysplasia (FMD).
57. A characteristic **"string-of-beads"** appearance on angiography is seen in cases of FMD.
58. FMD is typically located in the middle or distal third of the renal artery. In upto two-thirds (66.6%) of cases, it is bilateral. When unilateral FMD more commonly involves the **right artery**.
59. The most common **paediatric renovascular hypertension** is FMD.

Note: *Other cases are neurofibromatosis, the middle aortic syndrome, arteritis and William's syndrome.*

60. **"Cobra head deformity"** is seen on IVP in patients those who have ureterocoele.
61. The best way to visualize the **uterus and ovaries** in ultrasound (US).
62. **Renal angiography** is currently used only for selected indications like–
    - Evaluation and possible treatment (by baloon angioplasty) of renal artery stenosis.
    - For the treatment of renal haemorrhage by embolic occlusion of the bleeding renal artery branches.

63. **Male urethra** in children is best evaluated by doing a voiding cystourethrogram (VCUG). While in young adults a retrograde urethrogram is done to evaluate the male urethra.
64. Two situations (clinical) for which CYSTOGRAM study is indicated are possible rupture of the urinary bladder and urinary incontinence in a woman.
65. The **most sensitive radiologic test for urinary tract stones** are CAT scan, performed without contrast.

> ***Note:*** *Almost all types of urinary stones are visible on CAT scan.*

66. The **best initial imaging test for renal obstruction** is ultrasound.
67. A **nuclear renal scan** using either Tc-99m radioisotope or DTPA or mercaptoacetyltriglycine (MAG-3) is useful for monitoring the function of each kidney in patient with renal failure. It is accurate, relatively inexpensive and noninvasive.
68. The **best imaging modality for guiding renal biopsy** is ultrasound.
69. **Angiographic findings in renal artery stenosis** include—
    - Diameter of the aorta decreased by 50%.
    - Poststenotic dilatation.
    - Diminished ipsilateral renal size.
    - Diminished velocity of flow.
    - Collateral vessels.
    - Pressure gradient greater than 20% of peak systolic pressure.
70. The **best study for suspected gas forming infection in the urinary tract** is CAT scan.
71. **Enumerate the imaging findings of urinary tract infection (UTI) with tuberculosis:**
    - Findings are usually unilateral/asymmetric.
    - Renal abscess often with involvement of perinephric space and the psoas muscle (acute phase).

- Papillary necrosis.
- Stricture of the collecting system.
- Strictures of ureter which may have skip areas (**cock screw ureter**) or be continuous (**pipestem ureter**).
- Calcification in the kidney and proximal ureter.
- Calcifications in the perinephric space and psoas muscle.
- Shrunken, heavily calcified, nonfunctioning kidney (autonephrectomy).

72. The most common renal mass is renal simple cyst and the best way to confirm a renal mass is an ultrasound.
73. The most common **internist's tumour** is renal cell C_A.
74. The most common sarcoma of the kidney is **leiomyosarcoma**.
75. The most common renal malignancy of childhood is **Wilms' tumour**.
76. A radiologic tests useful in working up a patient who wants to donate a kidney for transplantation includes IVP Q renal angiography.
77. The imaging modalities most often used in the **evaluation of the adrenals** in CAT scan, MRI scan and in neonates ultrasound.
78. The **best initial radiologic test for evaluating the adrenals** is CAT scan.
79. Regarding the **rule of ten** (10) in respect of **pheochromocytomas**.
    - Bilateral in 10%.
    - Extradural in 10%.
    - Malignant in 10%.
    - Familial in 10%.

> ***Note:*** *Associated syndromes are easily remembered by the mnemonic: VEIN*
> *V : Von Hipple Lindau syndrome.*
> *E : Eudocrine neoplasm (in MEN type II).*
> *I : Inherited.*
> *N : Neurofibromatosis.*

80. Iodine^{131}–MIBG (Metaiodobenzyle Guanidine) is the nuclear agent of choice for detecting or

confirming the presence of a **phaeochromocytoma**.

81. **Neuroblastomas**, arise from the sympathetic nervous system, occur in children (very young) and are found in adrenal gland. These are malignant tumours.
82. The common imaging modalities used for **evaluation of scrotal diseases** are sonography, nuclear scintigraphy and MRI scan.
83. The most common type of testicular germ cell tumour is **seminoma**.
84. The **most aggressive type of testicular germ cell tumour** is embryonal cell carcinoma.
85. The **imaging test of choice in dealing with a palpable scrotal mass** in sonography.
86. The **most common metastatic testicular tumour** is lymphoma.
87. The imaging modality useful in estimating the weight of the prostate gland is CAT, MRI, transabdominal ultrasound and transrectal ultrasound.
88. The T_1-weighted images (MRI) are useful for demonstrating areas of postbiopsy haemorrhage and the status of the neurovascular bundles and for determining whether there is gross invasion into the periprostatic fat.
89. The **T_2-weighted images** (MRI scan) best demonstrate the zonal anatomy of the prostate. It is best for demonstrating lesions within the prostate.
90. The **prostatic capsule** is best seen on MRI (imaging) scan.
91. The most commonly used screening tests for prostate C_A is **digital rectal examination** and monitoring of prostatic specific antigen (PSA).
92. The most common site of haematogenous metastases from prostate is **bone**. The most commonly involved site is **pelvic bone** then → lumbar spine → femur, thoracic spine and least common ribs.
93. About 80% of bony metastasis from prostate is **osteoblastic**.

10

Oncology at a Glance

You Should Know

1. **X-rays and gamma (γ) rays** are used for the treatment of **deep seated tumours**.
2. **Stereotactic radiosurgery** is a form of **radiotherapy**.
3. **Stereotactic radiosurgery** is the administration of a focussed high dose of radiation to a precisely defined volume of tissue in a single treatment, usually using the **gamma knife**.

> ***Note:*** *This procedure can potentially achieve* ***tumour*** *(< 3 cm)* ***ablation*** *without any actual surgery.*

4. During **allopurinol** administration plasma concentration of uric acid gets reduced because the drug is a **xanthine oxidase inhibitors** but the level of xanthine and hypoxanthine in such individual gets increased.
5. A **monoclonal antibody against CEA labelled with Tc^{99m}** is now approved for imaging of cancers with increased level of CEA and has been found to be more sensitive and specific than CT scans in the detection of both resectable and nonresectable disease.
6. In **brachytherapy**, the radiation source is placed close to the tumour. This intracavitary approach is used for many gynaecologic or oral neoplasms and occasionally for breast cancer.
7. In **teletherapy,** supervoltage radiotherapy is usually delivered with a linear accelerator, as

this instrument permits more precise beam localization and avoids the complication of skin radiation toxicity.

8. Examples of **new approaches to minimize radiation** to surrounding tissues while maximizing radiation to the cancer include **three-dimensional conformal radiation therapy** (3DCRT) and **intensity modulated radiation therapy** (IMRT). Conventional radiation beams are of uniform intensity.
9. **IMRT's** beam intensity is modulated to produce maximum doses where desired and minimum radiation to nearby normal tissues.

> ***Note:*** *Improved outcomes have been seen in cases of prostatic* C_A *receiving IMRT.*

10. Currently, > **50%** of all patients having cancer receive **RT** during course of their illness.
11. **RT** is frequently the sole agent used with **curative intent** for tumours of – Larynx, oral cavity, pharynx, oesophagus, Cx uterine, vagina, prostate, skin, Hodgkin's disease and some tumours of the brain and spinal cord.
12. **Ibritumomab tiuresan** is the 1st radiolabelled antibody to be used for the treatment of cancer particularly relapsed low grade NHL.
13. The balanced mixture of **antioxidants** found in a diet rich in **fruit** and **vegetables** may be more important and more effective in reducing cancer risk than beta-carotene supplementation.
14. **Vitamin E supplementation** is more promising in preventing oxidants induced tumorogenesis.
15. **Retinoids** are the best studied tumour chemo-preventive agents. **NSAIDs** (especially Cox–2 inhibitors) and hormonal agents like **Tamoxifen, Raloxifene, Finasteride,** appear to have an important role in prevention of some tumours/ cancers/malignancy.
16. **Isotretinoin** has been shown to suppress **Leukoplakia**, a premalignant lesion of the

aerodigestive tract. A low dose isotretinoin has been found effective here.

17. **High doses of isotretinoin** may prevent the development of second primary tumours in patient with early epidermoid C_A (Scc) of the head and neck region.
18. Todate, there has been a significantly **higher rate** of **second primary tumour** formation in **smokers Vs former** impact of active smoking in 2nd primary tumour development.

> ***Note:*** *An interesting recent report suggests that NICOTINE may suppress the antigrowth effects of refinoids in lung cancer cells.*

19. **Three strategies** that have been proved to **prevent liver carcinogenesis** are vaccination against HBV, treatment of chronic active hepatitis 'C' with interferon and deletion of premalignant and latent malignant cells in the remnant livers of patients undergoing total resection of hepatocellular carcinomas.
20. The **Retinamide fenretinide** (4–HPR) is a potent apoptosis-inducing synthetic vitamin A analog with significant *in vitro* activity. Fenretinide appears to reduce the activity of TELOMERASE, which is important in lung carcinogenesis.
21. **Angiogenesis** (the growth of new blood vessels) is thought to be an essential component of the ability of tumours to invade locally and to metastasize from the primary tumour site.
22. **Tumour angiogenesis** is regulated by angiogenic stimulators like vascular endothelial growth factor (VEGF, the ligand for the VEGF receptor) and the newly described **inhibitors of angiogenesis**–ANGIOSTATIN AND ENDOSTATIN.
23. **Thalidomide** has been shown to have anti-angiogenic properties as well as other antitumour effects.

24. **Matrix metalloproteases** that are thought to be important in the ability of cancer cells to metastasize.
25. The most extensively treated disease with immunotherapeutic modalities is **malignant melanoma.**
26. In **tumourogenesis**, the genetic changes usually involve increased or abnormal expression or activity of certain genes called as PROTO-NCOGENES, deletion or inactivation of tumour suppress genes and defects in DNA repair enzymes.

> ***Note:*** *These genetic changes may ensue by point mutation, gene amplification, gene rearrangement, or epigenetic changes such as altered gene methylation.*

27. The moment the cell becomes malignant their growth kinetics are similar to those of normal cells but lack regulation.

> ***Note:*** *For unclear reasons, tumour growth kinetics follows a* ***GOMPERTZIAN CURVE.*** *It states that "As the tumour mass increases, the fraction of dividing cells declines". Thus by the time a cancer is large enough to be detected clinically, its growth fraction is often small.*

28. **Cancer cells proceed through the same cell-cycle stages as normal cycling cells:** **G1** (period of preparation of DNA synthesis), **S** (DNA synthesis), **G2** (tetraploid phase proceeding mitosis in which integrity of DNA replication is assessed and **M** (mitosis). Some non-cycling cells may remain in a **G0** or resting phase for long periods.
29. In **AML,** 3 environmental exposures increase the risks–chronic benzene (C_6H_6) exposure, radiation expsure and prior treatment with alkylating agents and topoisomerase inhibitors II (e.g. Doxorubicin and etoposide).

> ***Note:*** *CML, myelodysplasia and myeloproliferative syndromes may all evolve into AML.*

30. **Chromosome 11q23 abnormalities** are often seen in leukemias developing after exposure to topoisomerase II inhibitors.
31. Certain genetic anomalies seen with acute promyelocytic leukemia (APL-Fab M3) t (15; 17), inv (16) with eosinophilic variety.
32. In CML, over **90%** of cases have a reciprocal translocation between **chromosomes I and 22**, creating the **philadelphia** chromosome and a **fusion gene product** called **bcr–abl** (bcr is from 9, abl from 22).

> ***Note:*** *The chromosome abnormality appear in all bone-marrow derived cells except T cells.*

33. In CML cases, the protein made by chimeric gene is 210 kDa in chronic phase and 190 kDa in acute blast transformation.

> ***Note:*** *In some patient, the chronic phase is clinically silent and patients present with acute leukemia with the* ***philadelphia chromosome.***

34. In MDS (myelodysplastic syndrome), chromosome abnormalities ensue in upto 80% of cases, including deletion of part or all of chromosomes 5, 7, 9 (20 or 21 less commonly) and addition of part or all of chromosome 8.
35. The most common myeloproliferative syndrome is polycythemia rubra vera.

> ***Note:*** *Polycythemia rubra vera is the only ERYTHROCYTOSIS condition in which the ERYTHROPOIETIN level is low.*

36. In lymphoid malignancies, some genetic alterations are characteristics like t (8; 14) in Burkitt's lymphoma, t (14, 18) in follicular lymphoma, t (11; 14) in mantle cell lymphoma, t (2, 5) in anaplastic large cell lymphoma, translocations or mutations involving bcl-6 on 3q 27 in diffuse large cell lymphoma and others.

> **Note:** *In most cases, translocations involve insertion of a distant chromosome segment into the antigen receptor genes (either Ig Tcell receptor) during the rearrangement of the gene segments that form the receptors.*

37. Three viruses, EBV, HHV–8 and HTLV–I (a retrovirus) may cause some lymphoid malignancies.
38. EBV has been strongly associated with African's Burkitt's lymphoma and the lymphomas that complicate immune deficiencies.

> **Note:** *EBV has an uncertain relationship to mixed cellularity Hodgkin's disease and angiocentric lymphoma.*

39. Human herpesvirus–8 (HHV–8) causes a rare **"Body cavity lymphoma"** mainly in patients with AIDS. HTLV–1 is associated with adult T cell leukemia/lymphoma.

> **Note:** *Both HHV–8 and HTLV–1 diseases are endemic to South Western Japan and Caribbean Islanders.*

40. Gastric *Helicobacter pylori* infection is associated with gastric MALT lymphoma and perhaps gastric large cell lymphoma.
41. Inherited or acquired immunodeficiencies and antoimmune disorders predispose individual to lymphoma.
42. **Lymphoma** occurs with increased incidence in **farmers** and **meat workers.**
43. Incidence of Hodgkin's disease is increased in **wood workers**.
44. Follicular centre lymphoma is the most common indolent lymphomas accounting for about one-third of all lymphoid malignancies.
45. In follicular lymphoma, the t(14; 18) is present in 85% of cases resulting in the over expression of bcl–2, a protein involved in prevention of programmed cell death.

46. Follicular lymphoma cells also have a high rate of mutation that leads to the accumulation of genetic damage. Overtime, such lymphoma acquire sufficient genetic damage (e.g. mutated p53) to accelerate their growth and evolve into diffuse large cell lymphomas that are refractory to treatment.
47. In ALL, prognosis is adversely affected by high presenting WBC count, age >35 years and the presence of t(9; 22), t(1; 19) and t (4, 11) translocations (FABL1 children, FABL2 adults).
48. Burkitt's lymphoma is more common in children. It is associated with translocations involving the c-myc gene on chromosome 8 rearranging with Ig heavy or light chain genes.

> **Note:** *If leukemic picture predominates, then classified as FABL3.*

49. Regarding **plasma cell disorders**—
    - The hallmark is the production of Ig molecules or fragments from abnormal plasma cells.
    - The intact Ig mol or the heavy or light chain produced by the abnormal plasma cell clone, is detectable in the serum and/or urine is called M (monoclonal) component.
    - The amount of M component in any given patient reflects the tumour burden in that patient.
    - In some, the presence of a clonal light chain in the urine (Bence Jones protein) is the only tumour product that is detectable.

> **Note:** *M component may be seen in patients with other lymphoid tumours, nonlymphoid cancers, and noncancerous conditions like cirrhosis, sarcoidosis, parasitic infestations and autoimmune diseases.*

50. Multiple myeloma is a malignant transformation of plasma cells in bone marrow only not in lymph nodes.

51. The diagnostic triad of multiple myeloma includes bone marrow plasmacytosis > 10%, lytic bone lesions and a serum and/or urine M component.
52. **Regarding Hodgkin's disease (HD)**–
    - HD is a tumour of Reed-Sternberg cells, aneuploid cells that usually express CD30 and CD15 but may also express other B or T cell markers.
    - Most tumours are derived from B cells in that Igs genes.
    - About 85% cases are curable.
53. **Regarding skin cancers**–
    - **Malignant melanoma**–the most dangerous skin tumour.
    - MM may associated with **9p** deletion.
    - Superficial spreading melanoma is the most common type of MM.
    - Acral lentiginous is most common in darkly pigment MM patients.
    - **Basal cell C_A** (BCC) the most common and most frequent skin cancer on sun exposed skin (face).
    - **Noduloulcerative** (BCC) is the most common of the five variety.
    - Predisposing to BCC includes– fair complexion, exposure to UV light, and inorganic arsenicals like Fowler's solution or Paris green and ionizing radiation.
    - **Squamous cell C_A** (SCC) or epidermoid C_A is seen in fair complexion, chronic UVL exposure, previous burn or other scars, and exposure to inorganic arsenic or radiation.
    - **Actinic Keratosis** is a premalignant lesion.
    - SCC most commonly seen as ulcerated nodule or superficial erosion of skin.
    - Three types of SCC_A includes Bowen's disease, Scar C_A and verrucous C_A–seen most commonly on plantar aspect of foot.
54. Patient who have survived head and neck C_A commonly develop 2nd cancer of the head and

neck, lung, or oesophagus, presumably reflecting the exposure of the upper aerodigestive mucosa to similar carcinogenic stimuli.

55. In head and neck tumours, chromosomal deletions and mutations have been found in chromosomes 3p, 9p, 17p, 11q, and 13q and mutations in p53 have been reported.

> ***Note:*** *Cyclin D1 may be over expressed.*

56. In head and neck malignancy, locally advanced disease is the most common c/p and surgery with radiotherapy is the choice treatment.
57. Patient with head and neck C_A who are rendered disease free may benefit from chemopreventive therapy with cis-retinoic acid.
58. **Lung C_A** cells may have ≥ 10 aquired genetic lesions, most commonly point mutations in ras oncogenes; amplification, rearrangement, transcriptional activation of myc oncogenes, overexpression of bcl–2, Her–2/neu, and telomerase. Deletions involving chromosomes 1p, 1q, 3p 12–13, 3p14, (FHIT inhibitors), 11p13, 11p15, 13q14 (rb gene), 16q, and 17p13 (p53 gene).
    - Lung to lung metastaše is seen in Adeno C_A lung.
    - Lung is the most common site of metastasis.

> ***Note:***
> *i. Loss of 3p and 9p are the earliest events, detectable even in **hyperplastic bronchial epithelium.***
> *ii. p53 abnormalities and ras point mutations are usually found only in **invasive cancers.***

59. All patients of lung C_A are subjected to radiotherapy (RT) for brain metastases, spinal cord compression, weight bearing lytic bony lesions, symptomatic local lesions (nerve palsy, obstructed airway, hemoptysis in non-small cell lung C_A and in small cell C_A not responding to chemotherapy.

60. **Regarding breast C_A–**

- Most common tumour among women in the Western World (USA).
- Men also get breast C_A at the rate of **150 : 1**.
- It is hormone dependent.
- Women with late menarche, early menopause, and 1st full term pregnancy by age 18 have a significantly reduced risk.
- Women who received therapeutic radiation before age 30 are at incresed risk.
- Risk is increased in woman whose mother and sister also have had breast C_A. Perhaps 8 to 10% are familial.
- BRCA-1 mutation accounts for 5% while BRCA-2 chromosome 11 may account for 2 to 3% of breast C_A.
- BRCA-1 maps to chromosome 17q21 and appears to be involved in transcription-coupled DNA repair.

> ***Note:*** *The BRCA-1 syndrome includes an increased risk of ovarian C_A and prostatic C_A in women and men respectively.*

- Germline mutations in p53 (Li-Fraumeni syndrome) are very rare, but breast C_A, sarcomas, and other malignancies occur in such families.

> ***Note:*** *Sporadic breast C_A show many genetic alterations including overexpression of HER-2/neu in 25% of cases, p53 mutations in 40% and loss of heterozygosity at other loci.*

- Expression of oestrogen receptor improves prognosis, while overexpression of HER-1/neu, mutation in p53, high growth fraction and aneuploidy worsen the prognosis.
- Breast C_A can spread almost anywhere but commonly goes to bone, lungs, liver, soft tissues and brain.
- Breast C_A will recur in 50% of cases with localized disease.

- Patients with locally advanced breast C_A benefit from neoadjuvant chemotherapy that includes an anthracycline (CAF) followed by surgery plus breast radiation therapy (RT).

61. **Regarding GIT tumours–**

A. *Oesophageal C_A–*

- Male predominance.
- Highest incidence in focal regions of China, Iran, Afghanistan, Siberia, Mangolia.
- In USA, Blacks affected more than Whites.
- Presents in 6th decades or later, 5-year survival < 5% because most patients present with advanced disease.
- SCC (60%) most commonly seen in upper two-thirds.
- Adeno C_A (< 40%) seen in lower (distal) one-third arises from **Barrett's** oesophagus.
- Major risk factors include (for SCC)– Alcohol abuse, Tobacco smoking chronic ingestion of extremely hot tea/coffee. Deficiency of vitamin A, Zinc and Molybdenum. Others lye ingestion and oesophageal stricture, achalasia, radiation exposure, head and neck C_A, smoked opiates, plummer vinson syndrome, and Tylosis.
- Most sensitive and specific test is flexible oesophagogastroscopy.

B. *Gastric C_A*

- Highest incidence in Japan, Chile, China and Ireland.
- Incidence decreasing worldwide, Male female = 2:1.
- Peak incidence 6th and 7th decades. Overall 5 year survival < 15%.
- Increased incidence in low social group. Dietary factors-nitrates smoked foods, heavily salted foods, 1st degree relatives of affected patients. Other factors-

atrophic gastritis, *Helicobacter pylori* Billroth II gastrectomy, gastrojejunostomy, adenomatous gastric polyps, pernicious anemia, hyperplastic gastric polyps, Menetrier's disease, slight increased risk with blood group 'A' individual.

> ***Note:*** *Pernicious anaemia and hyperplastic gastric polyps are associated with* ***Atrophic gastritis.***

- Adeno CA (85%) usually focal (polypoid, ulcerative), two-thirds arising in **antrum** or **lesser curvature**, frequently ulcerative (intestinal type) less commonly diffuse infiltrative (limit is plastica) or superficial spreading (diffuse lesions more prevalent in younger patient and have extremely poor prognosis).
- Supraclavicular lymphadenopathy (Virchow's node, Troisier's sign).
- Periumbilical, ovarian or prerectal mass (Blummer's shelf).
- Acanthosis nigricans and dermatomyositis, multiple seborrheic keratosis.
- Iron deficiency anemia in two-thirds of patients and occult blood positive in 80%.
- Gastroscopy is the choice investigation allowing visualisation, biopsies and cytology.
- Low grade MALT lymphoma is caused by *H. pylori* infection.

C. *Hereditary Polyposis Syndrome (HPS)*

i. ***Familial Polyposis Coli (FPC)***

- Diffuse pancolonic adenomatous polyposis (upto several thousand polyps).
- Autosomal dominant inheritance associated with deletion in APC gene on chromosome 5.
- Colon CA from malignant degeneration of polyp in 100% by age 40.

> ***Note:*** *Sulindac and other NSAIDs cause regression and stop their development.*

ii. ***Gardner's syndrome***
- Variants of FPC with associated soft tissue tumours (osteomas, epidermoid cysts, lipomas, fibromas, desmoids etc).
- Higher incidence of gastroduodenal polyps.
- Ampullary adenocarcinoma.

iii. ***Turcot's syndrome***
- Rare variant of FPC with associated malignant brain tumours.

iv. ***Non-polyposis syndrome***
- Familial syndrome with upto 50% risk of colonic C_A.
- Peak incidence in 5th decade.
- Associated with multiple primary cancers especially endometrial C_A.
- Autosomal dominant.
- Due to defective DNA repair.

v. ***Juvenile polyposis***
- Multiple benign colonic and small bowel hamartomas.
- Intestinal bleeding common.
- Other symptoms: abdominal pain, diarrhoea, occasional intususception.
- Rarely recur after excision.
- Low risk of colon C_A from malignant degeneration of interspersed adenomatous polyps.

vi. ***Peutz-Jeghers syndrome***
- Numerous hamartomatous polyps of entire GIT tract though denser in small bowel than colon.
- GIT bleeding common.
- Somewhat increased risk for the development of cancer at GIT and non- GIT sites.

D. *Colorectal carcinoma*
- Most colon C_A arises from adenomatous polyps.

- Genetic steps from polyp to dysplasia to C_A in *situ to* invasive C_A have been defined, including: Point mutation, in K-ras proto-oncogene, hypomethylation of DNA leading to enhanced gene expression, allelic loss at the APC gene (a tumour suppressor), allelic loss at the DCC (deleted in colon C_A) gene on chromosome 18 and loss of mutation of p53 on chromosome 17.
- Hereditary nonpolyposis colon C_A arises from mutations in the DNA mismatch repair genes, hMSH2 gene on chromosome 2 and MLHI gene on chromosome 3.
- Mutation lead to colon and other cancers.
- **Diagnosis** requires three or more relatives with colon C_A, one of whom is a 1st degree relative, one or more cases diagnosed before age 50 and involvement of at least two generations.
- Environmental factors also play a role, increased prevalence in developed nation, urban areas, advantaged socioeconomic groups.
- Increased risks in patients with hyper-cholesterolemia, coronary artery disease, correlation of risks with low fibre, high animal fat diet.
- **Decreased risk** with long-term dietary Ca^{++} supplementation, daily ASPIRIN ingestion.
- **Increased risk** in 1st degree relatives of patients, families with increased prevalence of cancer, and patient with history of breast or gynaecologic C_A, familial polyposis syndromes, > 10-year history of ulcerative colitis or Crohn's disease (colitis), > 15 years history of ureterosigmoidostomy.
- Tumour in patient with story F/H of malignancy are frequently located in right colon and commonly present before age 50.

- High prevalence in patient having ***Streptococcus bovis*** bacteremia.
- Almost always adeno C_A.
- 75% located in distal to splenic flexure except in association with polyposis or hereditary cancers syndromes may be polypoid, sessile, fungating, constricting.
- Degree of invasiveness at surgery (Duke's classification) is single best predictor of prognosis.

> **Note:** *Rectosigmoid tumours may spread to lungs early because of systemic paravertebral venous drainage of this area.*

- Predictors serum CEA > 5 ng/ml or > 5 μg/L.
  - Poorly differentiated histology.
  - Bowel perforation.
  - Venous invasion.
  - Adherence to adjacent organs.
  - Aneuploidy.
  - Specific deletions in chromosomes 5, 17, 18 and mutation of ras proto-oncogene.
  - 15% have defects in DNA repair.

> **Note:** *Early detection of colonic C_A may be facilitated by routine screening of stool for occult blood.*

E. *Anal Carcinoma*

- Associated with chronic irritation, e.g. from condyloma acuminata, perianal fissures/ fistulae, chronic haemorrhoids or piles, leukoplakia, trauma from anal intercourse (sodomy).
- Women are more commonly affected than men.
- Homosexual men are at increased risk.
- Presents with bleeding, pain and perianal mass.
- Lesions < 3 cm responds well to radiotherapy + 5FU + mitomycin.

- Large lesion needs abdominoperineal resection.

F. *Hepatic Tumours*

i. ***Benign Hepatic Tumours***

- Seen most commonly in women in the 3rd or 4th decades who uses OCPs.
- Most are diagnosed incidentally but may cause pain, intratumoral haemorrhage may cause circulatory collapse (**Shock**).
- 10% may become malignant.

> **Note:** *It is mandatory that women harbouring such adenomas should stop using birth control pills (OCPs).*

ii. ***Hepatocellular C_A or Hepatoma***

- Tumour usually develops in cirrhotic liver in persons in 5th or 6th decade. Male female ratio being 4:1.
- High incidence in Asia and Africa owing to its relationship with HBV and HCV infections.
- Aflatoxin exposure contributes to aetiology and a mutation in codon 249 of this gene for p53.
- Hepatitis 'B' vaccine prevents the disease.

> **Note: Interferon** *a-may prevent liver C_A in persons with CAH 'C' disease and possibly in those with hepatitis 'B'.*

G. *Pancreatic cancer*

> **Note:** *Nearly all diagnosed pancreatic C_A are fatal because it is not diagnosed until the disease has spread.*

- The tumour is ductal adeno-C_A and about 70% seen in head, 20% in body and 10% in pancreatic tail.
- **Mutations** in **K-ras** have been found in 85% of tumours, and the **P16 cyclin depen-**

dent kinase inhibitor on **chromosome I** may also be implicated.

- Long-standing DM, chronic pancreatitis, and smoking increase the risk. But coffee drinking, alcoholism and cholelithiasis do not.
- Patient present with pain and weight loss.

> ***Note:*** *The pain often relieved by bending forward.*

- **Jaundice** commonly complicates tumours of the head, due to biliary obstruction.
- GEMCITABINE may palliate symptoms in patients with advanced disease.

H. *Endocrine Tumours of GIT*

i. ***Carcinoid Syndrome***

- Accounts for 75% of GIT endocrine tumours.
- Incidence 15 cases per million.
- 90% arises from kulchitsky cells of the GIT.
- Most common seen in appendix, ileum and rectum.

> ***Note:*** *Carcinoid tumours of the small bowel and bronchus have a more malignant course than tumours of other sites.*

- About 5% of patients with carcinoid tumours develop symptoms of carcinoid syndrome, the **classic triad** being cutaneous flushing, diarrhoea and valvular heart disease.
- For tumours of GIT origin, symptoms imply metastases to liver.
- Diagnosis can be made by detecting the site of tumour or documenting production of > 15 mg/day of the serotonin (5-HT) metabolite-5-hydroxy indole acetic acid (5-HIAA) in the urine.

> ***Note:*** *Octreotide scintigraphy identifies sites of primary and metastatic tumour in about two-thirds of cases.*

- Median survival of patients with carcinoid syndrome is 2.5 years from the 1st episode of flushing.

ii. ***Pancreatic islet cell tumours***

- Gastrinoma, insulinoma, VIPOMA, glucagonoma and somatostatinoma account for the vast majority of pancreatic islet cell tumours.
- These tumours are so named for the dominant hormone they produce.
- They are generally slow-growing and produce symptoms related to hormone production.
- **Gastrinomas** and peptic ulcer disease comprise the Zollinger-Ellison syndrome. These are rare and in 25 to 50%, the tumour is a component of MENI syndrome.
- **Insulinomas** may present with Whipple's triad, fasting hypoglycemia, symptoms of hypoglycemia and relief after I.V. glucose infusion.

> ***Note:*** *Normal or elevated serum insulin levels in presence of fasting hypoglycemia are diagnostic.*

- Insulinoma may also be associated with MENI.
- VIPOMA—**Verner** and **Morrison** described a syndrome of watery diarrhoea, hypokalemia (↓ K^+), achlorhydria, and renal failure associated with pancreatic islet cell tumour that produce VIP (vasoactive intestinal polypeptide).
- Vipomas are rare but often grows to large size before producing symptoms.
- **Glucagonoma** is associated with DM and necrolytic migratory erythema, a characteristic red, raised,scaly rash usually located on the face, abdomen, perineum and distal extremities.

> ***Note:*** *Glucagon levels > 1000 ng/L, not suppressed by glucose are diagnostic.*

- **Somatostatinoma**–The classic triad of somatostatinoma is DM, steatorrhoea and cholelithiasis.
- Provocative tests may facilitate diagnosis of functional endocrine tumours; Tolbutamide enhances somatostatin secretion by somatostatinomas.
- **Pentagastrin** enhances calcitonin secretion from medullary thyroid (C cell) tumours.
- **Secretin** enhances gastrin secretion from gastrinomas.
- If imaging techniques fail to detect tumour masses angiography or selective venous sampling for hormone determination may reveal the site of tumour.
- Metastases to nodes and liver should be sought by CT or MRI.

62. **Genitourinary Tract Cancer**

i. *C_A Bladder*

- Median age of occurrence is 65 years.
- Smoking accounts for 50% of risk.
- Exposure to polycyclic aromatic hydrocarbons increases the risk especially in slow acetylators.
- Greater risks seen in chimney sweepers, drycleaners and those associated with aluminium production.

> ***Note:***
> *i. Chronic cyclophosphamide exposure increases 9 fold risk.*
> *ii. **Schistosoma haematobium** infection also increases risk especially for **SCC** of urinary bladder.*

- Lesions involving chromosome 9q are an early event. Deletion in 17p (p53), 18q (the DCC locus), 13q (RB), 3p, and 5q are characteristic of invasive lesions.

- Overexpression of epidermal growth factor receptors and HER-2/neu receptors is common.
- More than 90% of tumours are derived from transitional epithelium only 3% SCC, and 20% are adeno C_A and < 1% are neuroendocrine small cell C_A.
- **Field effects** are seen that place all sites lined by transitional epithelium at risk including the renal pelvis, ureter, bladder and proximal two-thirds of the urethra.
- 90% of tumours are in the urinary bladder, 8% in the renal pelvis, and 2% in the ureter or urethra.
- Haematuria is the initial sign in 80 to 90%.

> **Note:** *Cystitis is the more common cause of haematuria (23%).*

- Intravesicle instillation of BCG reduces the risk of recurrence by 40 to 45%. Recurrence is monitored every 3 monthly.
- Standard treatment is radical cystectomy. But those who cannot tolerate it should be treated with radiotherapy 5000 to 7000 cG EBR.

ii. *Renal Carcinoma*

> **Note:** *Tobacco smoking accounts for 20 to 30% of cases.*

- Risk is increased in acquired renal cystic disease. There are two familial forms; a rare AD syndrome and Von Hipple-Lindau syndrome.

> **Note:** *About **35%** of Von-Hippel-Lindau disease develop renal C_A.*

- Incidence is also increased in tuberous sclerosis and polycystic kidney disease.
- The most frequent chromosomal abnormality seen in 60% of cases is deletion or rearrangement of 3p21-26.

- The Von-Hippel Lindau gene has been mapped to that region and appears to have novel activities, regulation of speed of transcription and participation in turnover of damaged protein.

> ***Note:*** *It is not clear how lesions in the gene produces cancer.*

- Five variants are recognized.
  - Clear cell tumours (75%).
  - Chromophilic tumours (15%).
  - Chromophobic tumours (5%).
  - Oncocytic tumours (3%).
  - Collecting duct tumours (2%).
- Clear cell tumours arise from cell of the proximal convoluted tubules.
- Chromophilic tumours tend to be bilateral and multifocal and often show trisomy 7 and/or trisomy 17.
- Chromophobic and eosinophilic tumours less frequently have chromosomal aberrations and follow a more indolent course.
- The **classic triad** of heamaturia, flank pain and flank mass seen only in 10 to 20% of cases, haematuria (40%), flank pain (40%), palpable mass (33%), weight loss (33%) are the most common individual symptoms.
- Paraneoplastic syndromes of RBCs (3%), hypercalcemia (5%) and iron metastatic hepatic dysfunction **(Stauffer's syndrome)** (15%), may also seen.
- Evaluation includes- urinalysis, cytology, X-ray, I.V. pyelography, renal ultrasonography, CT of abdomen and pelvis.
- **Stage I disease**—confined to kidney.
- **Stage II disease**—contained within Gerota's fascia.
- **Stage III disease**—locally invasive involving nodes and IVC.

- **Stage IV disease**—invasion of adjacent organ or metastatic site.
- Prognosis depends on staging—5-year survival rate for stage I (66%), stage II (64%), stage III (42%) and stage IV (11%).
- For stages I, II and III—Radical nephrectomy.

> **Note:** *About 10 to 15% of patient with advanced stage disease may benefit from* ***interleukin-2*** *and/or* ***interferon-a****.*

iii. *Testicular Carcinoma or (C_A Testis)*

- Peak incidence–20 to 40 years.
- Occurs 4 to 5 times more frequently than blacks.
- Cryptorchid (undescended) testis are at increased risk.

> **Note:** *Early orchidopexy may protect feminization syndromes and Klinefelter's syndrome (mediastinal germ cell variety).*

- Disease is associated with a characteristic cytogenetic defect **isochromosome 12p**.
- Pathologically two main types—
  i. Seminoma.
  ii. Non-seminoma.
- **Seminoma** has a more indolent natural history (N/H) and is highly sensitive to **radiotherapy**.
- **Non-seminoma**–4 subtypes described—
  a. Embryonal C_A.
  b. Teratoma.
  c. Choriocarcinoma.
  d. Endodermal sinus (Yolk sac) tumour.
- C/P-**Painless** testicular mass-classic sign.

> **Note :** *Painful testicular mass - epididymitis/or orchitis.*

- **Evaluation** needs-estimation of α-fetoprotein and β-hCG. X-ray chest, CT scan—abdomen and pelvis.

> **Note:** *hCG is elevated in either seminoma or nonseminoma but a-feto-protein (AFP) is elevated in nonseminoma only.*

63. **Gynaecologic Cancer.**

i. *Ovarian Tumour/Cancer.*

- Incidence begins to rise in 5th decade, peak in 8th decade.

> **Note:** *Risk is increased in nulliparous women and reduced by pregnancy (risk decreased about 10% per pregnancy) and oral contraceptives.*

- About 5% familial.
- **Mutations** in BRCA-1 predispose women to both breast and ovarian cancer.
- Cytogenetic analysis of epithelial ovarian cancers that are not familial often reveals complex karyotypic abnormalities including structural lesions on chromosomes I and II and loss of heterozygosity for loci on chromosomes 3q, 6q, 11q, 13q and 17q.
- C-myc, H-ras, K-ras and HER^2/neu are often mutated or overexpressed.
- Adrenal masses in postmenopausal women are more often pathologic and should be surgically removed.
- C_A-125 serum levels are ≥ 35 u/ml in 80 to 85% of women with ovarian C_A.

> **Note:** *CEA elevation also seen in others.*

- Malignant ovarian tumours (33.3%) may be of 6 types–
  a. Serous–50%
  b. Clear cell–5%
  c. Mucinous–25%
  d. Brenner tumours–1% (urothelial or Transitional)
  e. Endometrioid–15%
  f. Stromal/germ cell–4%.

- Advanced stage patient should received **paclitaxel**, 175 mg/m^2 by 3h-infusion, followed by **carboplastin** dosed to an area under the curve (AUC) of 7.5 every 3 or 4 weeks.

> ***Note:*** *Carboplastin dose is calculated by the* ***calvert formula****.*
> *Calvert formula:*
> *dose = target AUC × (GFR + 25).*

- The complete response rate is about 55%, and median sruvival is 38 months.

ii. *Endometrial C_A.*

> ***Note:*** *The most common gynaecologic C_A in USA.*

- It is primarily a disease of postmenopausal ladies.
- Obesity, altered menstruation, infertility, late menopause, and postmenopausal bleeding are commonly encountered in women with this cancer.
- Women taking oestrogen replacement therapy and using tamoxifen for preventing breast C_A recurrence are at a modestly increased risk.
- Peak incidence seen in 6th and 7th decades.
- Abnormal vaginal discharge (90%), abnormal vaginal bleeding (80%) and leukorrhoea (10%) are the most common symptoms.
- These are adeno C_A in 75 to 80% of cases.
- **Prognosis** depends on stage, histologic grade, and degree of myometrial invasion.
- Total abdominal hysterectomy and bilateral salpingo-oophorectomy comprise both the staging procedure and treatment of choice.

iii. *CA Cervix*

- It is the commonest genital cancer among women in India and other developing nations having low social status (economic).

- Women having early sexual activity, multiple sexual partner and in cigarette (tobacco) smokers.
- HPV types 16 and 18 are the major types associated with C_AC_X.

> **Note:** *The HPV attacks the G1 checkpoint of the cell cycle, it* ***E7*** *protein binds and inactivates Rb protein, and* ***E6*** *induces the degradation of* ***P53****.*

- If there is evidence of C_A *in situ* during screening for C_AC_X a cone biopsy is performed, which is therapeutic.
- **Stage I** disease is treated with radical hysterectomy or radiotherapy.
- **Stage II to IV** diseases are usually treated with radiotherapy often with both brachytherapy and teletherapy or combined modality therapy.
- Women with locally advanced (Stage II B to IV A) disease usually receive concurrent chemotherapy and radiotherapy.

> **Note:** *The role of chemotherapy is to act as a radiosensitizer.*

- **Hydroxyurea, 5-FU** and **cisplatin** have all shown promising results given concurrently with radiotherapy.

iv. *Prostatic Hyperplasia*

> **Note:** *It is an universal finding in aging men, starting after 45 years and produces urinary outflow obstruction.*

- As the obstruction progresses, urinary stream caliber and force diminish, hesitancy in stream initiation develops, and postvoid dribbling ensues.

> **Note:** *Dysuria and urgency are sign of bladder irritation and usually not seen in prostatic hyperplasia.*

- On P/R examination-A hyperplastic prostate is smooth, firm and rubbery. The median groove may be lost.
- PSA elevated ≤ 10 ng/ml.
- Treatment-TUR (surgery).
- Drugs-Terazosin and Finasteride is used to reduce its size.

> ***Note:*** *Recently Transurethral Microwave Thermotherapy (TUMT) may be used which is equal to TUR surgery.*

v. *Prostatic* C_A

- More than 95% are **adeno** $\mathbf{C_A}$. It is more common in black.
- Although these patients show all clinical features of hyperplastic prostate but associated dysuria, back pain and hip pain are common.
- Biologic behaviour affected by histologic grade (Gleason score).
- It arises in periphery of gland and detectable on P/R examination as hard, irregular nodules.
- PSA elevated > 10 ng/ml. PSA level also correlates with spread, only 10% of those with PSA < 10 ng/ml have lymphatic spread. **Bone** is the most common site of distant metastases.
- Lymphatic spread is assessed surgically, it is present only in 10% of those with gleason grade 5 or lower and in 70% of those with grade 9 or 10.
- **WHITMORE-JEWETT staging** includes–
  a. Tumour not palpable but detected at TUR.
  b. Palpable tumour in one (B_1) or both (B_2) lobes.
  c. Palpable tumour outside capsule.
  d. Distant metastases.

Treatment: For patients of A to C disease-TUR or radiotherapy have claimed to be equal in response but TUR or surgery is preferred.

> ***Note:*** *Both surgery/radiotherapy causes IMPOTENCY.*

- Patients treated surgically for localized disease who develop rising PSA may undergo PROSTASCINT SCANNING.
- For patient with metastatic disease, ANDROGEN DEPRIVATION is the treatment of choice. Surgical castration is effective but most patient prefer to take LEUPROLIDE and FLUTAMIDE.

> ***Note:*** *Alternative approaches include adrenalectomy, hypophysectomy, oestrogen administration and medical adrenalectomy with aminoglutethimide.*

- The median survival of stage D patients is 33 months.
- Chemotherapy treated patients are more likely to have pain relief than those receiving supportive care alone.
- Bone pain from metastases may be palliated with **Strontium-89** or **Samarium-153**.

64. **Bone and Soft tissue Sarcomas**

i. *Soft Tissue Sarcomas*

- About 60% arise in extremities, lower: upper = 3:1, 30% on the trunk, often the retroperitoneum, 10% in the head and neck region.

> ***Note:*** *Sarcomas occur with increased frequency in persons who have undergone radiotherapy, who are immunosuppressed, (congenital or acquired) or those exposed to chemical carcinogen like polycyclic hydrocarbons, asbestos, and dioxin.*

- Sarcoma rarely develops within a scar from a prior operation, burn, injury, or foreign body implantation.
- **Kaposi's sarcoma** (a vascular tumour) is associated with **HSV 8** infection.
- Individuals with germline mutations in the P53 gene (Li-Fraumeni syndrome) are at increased risk for these and other malignancies.

> ***Note:*** *Those who have survived congenital Retinoblastoma (germline mutations in Rb gene) are at risk of developing sarcomas.*

- Such tumours spread haematogenously. **Lung** is the most common site.
- About twenty different types of sarcomas have been recognized based upon the normal tissue from which they originate like fibrous tissue, feet, skeletal/smooth muscles and blood vessels.
- Diagnosis is done by incisional biopsy.
- Imaging of primary tumour is best with plain x-ray and MRI scan for extremities and head neck lesions.

> ***Note:*** *CT scan is used for truncal lesions.*

- Stage I - well differentiated (75%).
- Stage II - intermediate differentiated (55%).
- Stage III - poorly differentiated (29%).
- Stage IV - patients with metastases present (< 20%).
- **Prognosis** is related to staging of the disease, five years survival rate is given above with stage.
- **Treatment** - Radical excision with documented histologic negative margins is the treatment of choice.
- Besides adjuvant radio/chemotherapy improve local control and permit the use

of a limb-sparing surgical procedure. Combination chemotherapy with doxorubicin and ifosfamide is used in the setting of metastatic disease and may cure 10 to 15% of patients.

ii. *Bone Sarcomas*

> **Note:** *Multiple myeloma is the commonest bone neoplasm.*

- Osteosarcoma, chondrosarcoma, Ewing's sarcoma and malignant fibrous histiocytoma are the major sarcomas involving bone.
- Benign bone tumours like enchondromas and osteochondromas may transform into chondrosarcoma and fibrous dysplasia and Paget's disease into osteosarcoma or malignant fibrous histiocytoma.

A. **Osteosarcoma (OS)**

- OS accounts for about 45% of bone sarcomas. 60% of OS occur in children and adolescents.
- Males are affected 1.5 to 2 times more frequently than females.
- OS has a predilection for the metaphyses of long bones, especially the distal femur and proximal tibia and humerus.

> **Note:** *Malignant fibrous histiocytoma is considered part of the spectrum of OS.*

- Patients present with pain and swelling in the affected area.
- Plain X-ray reveals–a destructive lesion with a moth-eaten appearance, a spiculated periosteal reaction **(Sun burst appearance)**, and a cuff of periosteal new bone formation at the margin of the soft tissue mass (called **Codman's triangle**).
- The disease is **radioresistant**.
- The standard treatment approach includes pre/post-operative chemotherapy with

doxorubicin, ifosfamide, cisplatin, high dose methotrexate along with limb spaning surgery.

B. **Chondrosarcoma (CS)**

- CS accounts for about 25% of all bone sarcomas.
- Peak incidence 4th or 6th decades of life.
- It has a predilection for flat bones the girdles (shoulder/pelvic).
- Radiologically, CS appear lobular with mattled, punctate or annular calcification.

> ***Note:*** *Chondrosarcomas (CS) are difficult to distinguish from benign cartilage tumours radiologically.*

- Clinical signs of progressive tumour growth and inflammation favour the malignant diagnoses.
- This neoplasm is resistant to chemotherapy.
- Surgery is the treatment of choice.

C. **Ewing's sarcoma (ES)**

- It accounts for 10 to 15% of bone sarcomas, chiefly seen in teenagers.
- ES has predilection for the diaphyses of long bones and for flat bones.
- Radiologically exhibits a characteristic **"onion peel periosteal reaction"** with a soft tissue mass.
- The tumour consists of sheets of small, round, blue staining cells that may be confused with lymphoma, small cell lung cancer, or embryonal rhabdomyosarcoma.
- The diagnosis is confirmed by detecting 30/32 product of the mic-2 gene on the cell surface.
- ES is a family member of such tumour called primitive neuro-ectodermal tumours (PNETs) occurring mostly in soft tissues.

> ***Note:*** *The characteristic chromosomal translocations associated with PNETs including ES is t(11; 22), which creates a chimeric gene product with components from the fli-1 gene on chromosome 11 and ews on 22.*

- The disease commonly spread to lungs, other bones and bone marrow.
- Systemic chemotherapy with doxombicin, ifosfamide, etoposide and vincristine is effective treatment and usually employed before limb spairing surgery.
- Peripheral primary lesions (below the elbow and mid-calf) have a 5 years survival of 80%.

> ***Note:*** *Even with metastastic disease, 25 to 40% are enable with high-dose radiotherapy and stem cell transplantation.*

65. **Cancer of Unknown Primary Site (COUPS)**
    - COUPS is defined as "Biopsy proven malignancy, primary site unapparant after history, physical exam, X-ray chest, abdomen and pelvis CT, CBC, chemistry survey, mammography (women), β-hCG level (men), α-fetoprotein levels, PSA level (men) and histologic evaluation not consistent with a primary tumour at the biopsy site.
    - COUPS incidence is gradually declining owing to better diagnostic pathologic sense. They now-a-days account for just 3% of all cancers. Most patients are > 60 years of age.
    - Cell line derived from such tumours frequently have abnormalities in **chromosome 1**.
    - **C/P** patients may present with fatigue, weight loss, pain, bleeding, abdominal swelling, subcutaneous masses, and lymphadenopathy.
    - In general, efforts to evaluate the presence of these tumour types depend more on the **pathologists** than on expensive clinical diagnostic testing.

- The careful L/M, E/M (ultrastructure) immunologic, Karyotypic and molecular biologic examination of adequate volumes of tumour tissues is the most important feature of the diagnostic workup in the absence of suspicious findings on history and physical examination.
- **Histopathology**–About 60% of COUPS are adeno C_A, SCC (10 to 20%), Rest 20 to 30% not further classied on L/M findings.
- **Prognosis**–Patients with SCC have median survival of 9 months and those with adeno C_A of 4 to 6 months.

> ***Note:*** *Patients in whom primary site is identified usually have a better outcome.*

Treatment: Patients without a primary diagnosis should be treated palliatively with RT to symptomatic lesions.

66. **Syndrome of Unrecognized extragonadal germ cell neoplasms**
    - In patients < 50 years with tumour involving midline structures, lung parenchyma or lymph nodes and evidence of rapid tumour growth, germ cell tumour is a possible diagnosis.
    - Serum tumour marker's may or may not be elevated.
    - **Cisplatin, etoposide, bleomycin,** chemotherapy may induce complete responses in ≥ 25% and ~15% may be cured.

> ***Note:*** *A trial of such therapy should also be undertaken in patients whose tumours have abnormalities in* ***chromosome 12.***

67. **Peritoneal carcinomatosis in women**
    - Women who presents with pelvic mass or pain and an adeno C_A diffusely throughout the peritoneal cavity, but without a clear site of origin, have primary peritoneal papillary serous C_A.

- The presence of **psammoma bodies** in the tumour or **elevated CA–125** levels may favour ovarian origin.
- Such patient should undergo debulking surgery followed by **paclitaxel** plus **cisplatin** combination therapy.

> ***Note:*** *About 20% responded to such therapy and 10% would survive for 2 years atleast.*

68. **CA axillary lymph node in women**
    - Such women should receive adjuvant breast C_A therapy appropriate for their menopausal status even in the absence of a breast mass on clinical examination or mammography and undetermined or negative oestrogen and progesterone receptors on the tumour.
    - Unless the ipsilateral breast is radiated, upto 50% of these patients will later develop a breast mass.
    - Although this is a rare clinical situation, long-term survival similar to women with stage II breast C_A is possible.
69. **Osteoblastic bone metastasis in men**
    - The possibility here of prostatic C_A is high. A trial of empirical hormonal therapy (Leuprolide and flutamide) is warranted.
70. **Cervical lymph node metastases**
    - Even if panendoscopy fails to reveal a head and neck primary, treatment of such patient with cisplatin and 5-FU treatment may be responsive.
    - Some responses are long lived.
71. **Pathologic evaluation of biopsy specimens from patients with metastatic cancer of unknown primary site.**

Evaluation/findings	*Suggested primary site/neoplasm*
1. **Histopathology (H and E stain)**	
• Psammoma bodies, papillary configuration.	Ovary/thyroid C_A.

Contd...

Contd...

Evaluation/findings	*Suggested primary site/neoplasm*
• Signet ring cells.	Stomach C_A.
2. **Immunohistology**	
• Leukocyte common antigen (LCA, CD45)	Lymphoid neoplasm.
• Leu-M1	Hodgkin's disease.
• Epithelial membrane antigen	C_A (Carcinoma)
• Cytokeratin intermediate fila-ments	C_A.
• CEA	C_A.
• HMB 45	Melanoma.
• Desmin	Sarcoma.
• Thyroglobulin	Thyroid C_A.
• Calcitonin	Medullary C_A thyroid.
• Myoglobin	Rhabdomyosarcoma.
• PSA/ prostatic acid phosphatase	Prostate.
• AFP	Liver, stomach, germ cell.
• Placental alkaline phosphatase	Germ cell.
• B, T cell markers	Lymphoid neoplasm.
• S-100 protein	Neuroendocrine tumour, melanoma.
• Gross cystic fluid protein	Breast, sweat gland.
• Factor VIII	Kaposi's sarcoma, angiosarcoma.
3. **Flow cytometry**	
• B,T, cell markers	Lymphoid neoplasm.
4. **E/M or ultrastructure**	
• Actin-myosin filaments	Rhabdomyosarcoma.
• Secretory granules	Neuroendocrine tumours.
• Desmosomes	C_A.
• Premelanosomes	Malanoma.
5. **Cytogenetics**	
• Isochromosome 12p; 12q(–)	Germ cell.
• t (11; 22)	Ewing's sarcoma, primitive neuroecto-dermal tumour.
• t (8; 14)	Lymphoid neoplasm.
• 3 p (–)	Small cell lung C_A, renal cell C_A, mesothelioma.
• t (X; 18)	Synovial sarcoma.
• t (12; 16)	Myxoid iposarcoma.

Contd...

Contd...

Evaluation/findings	*Suggested primary site/neoplasm*
• t (12; 22)	Clear cell sarcoma (Melanoma of soft parts).
• t (2; 13)	Alveolar rhabdomyosarcoma.
• 1 P (–)	Neuroblastoma.
6. **Receptor analysis**	
• Oestrogen/progesterone receptor	Breast.
7. **Molecular biologic studies**	
• I g, bcL-2, T-cell receptor gene rearrangement.	Lymphoid neoplasm.

11

Nuclear Medicine

You Should Know

1. Regarding a radionuclide used in scanning ideally should–
   - Emit no alpha (α) particles.
   - Emit no beta (β) particles.
   - Have no conversion electrons.
   - Have no very low-energy photons.
2. In a typical scanning device the greatest loss of efficiency is due to → GEOMETRY.
3. For RADIOIMMUNOASSAY the labeled hormone should–
   - Retain the ability to bind completely to the antibody.
   - Should not bind non-specifically to other serum proteins.
4. A **Radioisotopes** that can be released into sanitary sewage systems in a concentration greater than 100 μci (microcurie) per litre is → **^{99m}Technetium.**
5. A radionuclide that may produce pharmacologic effect in normally administered doses is 197 Mercury mercurohydrin.
6. Specific activity of a sample containing radioactive material is expressed by millicuries per gram.
7. The commonest brain tumour is → GLIOMA.
8. The greatest diagnostic accuracy of brain scanning is in → MENINGIOMA.
9. The ideal agent for CSF **scintigraphy** should maintain a high CSF to blood ratio.

10. The agent of choice for brain scanning is Technetium 99m- pertechnitate.
11. Three factors are important in identifying brain tumour during a brain scan–
    - Volume of the lesion.
    - Location within the brain.
    - Tumour brain radioactive concentration ratio.
12. Increased activity in a crescentic lateral distribution on the frontal scan, less prominently seen on the lateral scan, is found in–
    - Scalp trauma.
    - Subdural haematoma.
    - Pachymeningitis.
    - Paget's disease.
    - Post-craniotomy.
13. Pertechnetate as a brain scanning agent concentrates in the choroid plexus that causes confusion in interpretation and can be eliminated by prior oral administration of potassium perchlorate.
14. When scanning the vertex of the brain after the administration of pertechnetate large area of activity is seen as the result of nasal and oral mucous secretion that may be abolished by → **Atropine.**
15. The transverse sinuses on the normal posterior brain scan are usually asymmetrical with greater drain on the right.
16. Salivary gland scanning with Technetium 99m pertechnetate will give "hot" areas in → WARTHIN'S TUMOUR.
17. In differentiating Hashimoto's thyroiditis, multinodular goitre and carcinoma thyroid, thyroid scanning is not helpful.
18. The incidence of carcinoma in multinodular goitre is 1% only.
19. The commonest complication of radioiodide therapy for hyperthyroidism is → HYPOTHYROIDISM.
20. The normal range for thyroid uptake value is → 15 to 45%.

21. The factors that will not increase the radioiodine uptake is **dessicated thyroid**.
22. Recognised indications of radioiodine therapy in hyperthyroidism include:
    - Previous thyroidectomy for hyperthyroidism.
    - Exophthalmic goitre in persons over 25 years of age.
    - Long preoperative preparation.
    - Hyperthyroidism with surgical contraindications.
    - Hyperthyroidism with malignant exophthalmos.
23. The administration of TSH in a hypopituitary state is characterized by increased second uptake.
24. In the presence of conditions causing impaired iodination of TYROSINE such as thyroiditis, some cases of Graves' disease, a repeat 131 uptake following administration of perchlorate causes a marked drop in thyroid radioactivity.
25. The factors that decrease T_3 red cell uptake include:
    - Pregnancy.
    - Hepatitis.
    - Administration of Propylthiouracil.

> ***Note:*** *The factors do not decrease T_3 RBC uptake in Nephrosis.*

26. Recognized factors that do seriously elevate T_3 RBC uptake include–
    - Nephrosis.
    - Anticoagulant administration.
    - Administration of dilantin.
27. Less than 0.1% of the total circulating T_4 is "free".
28. The factors do not seriously elevate T_3 RBC uptake is → Administration of iodide.
29. To do a **thyroid uptake** study the normally administered dose of ^{131}I radioiodine is 5 µci (microcurie).

30. To do a **Thyroid scan** with ^{131}I Na^{I} (Sodium iodide), the dose given is normally about 25 μci (microcuries).
31. To do a **thyroid suppression test** prior to the second dose on ^{131}I Tri-iodothyronine (T_3) is given tds (three times) for 8 days.
32. The optimal size range for **human lung scanning** using ^{131}I macroaggregated albumin is 5 to 25 microns (μ).
33. In **lung scanning**, the lack of subjective symptoms or objective signs is due to the relatively small number of injected particles.
34. **Lung scans** should be done with no contrast enhancement.
35. Recognised mechanisms show diminished perfusion on **lung scans** include:
    - Alveolar hypoxia.
    - Organic blockage of pulmonary artery.
    - Extrapulmonic displacement of pulmonary tissue.
    - Pulmonary arterio-venous communication.
    - Bronchial artery–Pulmonary artery back flow.
    - Chronic pulmonary venous hypertension.
36. The absorbed radiation dose to the lungs from a 300 μci dose of ^{131}I macroaggregated is → 3 rads.
37. Usual cause of a "HOT" area seen on the lung scan using macroaggregated albumin is injection of the aggregate following blood clot formation within the syringe.
38. Perfusion **lung scans** done following bronchography will show new perfusion defects.
39. The most sensible and reliable test for **pericardial** effusion in the range of 200 to 300 cc of fluid is ULTRASONOGRAPHY.
40. To do a **renal scan**, the dose of 197 Mercury chlormerodrine is 1.5 μci per kg of body weight.
41. Doing a **renal scan** with 197 Mercury chlormerodrin, the dose to the renal cortex is **1 Rad**.

42. A **renal scan** should be done in **prone** position.
43. If the blood urea nitrogen (BUN) is over 100 mg percent **renal scanning** is best done with ^{131}I Hippuran.
44. The most reliable criterion for the diagnosis of unilateral renal vascular disease using radioisotope renography is the difference between the maximum amplitude of the curve minus the minimum amplitide of the curve.
45. In order to **scan the liver** with Technetium sulphur colloid, 2 millicuries is given intravenously.
46. The size of particles of ^{198}Au commonly used for **liver scanning** is 30 millimicrons.
47. The **highest radiation dose to the liver during liver scanning** with normal doses is given by ^{198}Au colloid.
48. A LIVER SCAN on a patient with advanced cirrhosis may show large cold areas due to–
    - Hepatoma.
    - Fatty replacement.
    - Fibrous replacement.
    - Portal-systemic vascular shunting.
49. In a patient with infiltration of the spleen by lymphoma or leukaemia, the **spleen scan** shows decreased splenic sequestration.
50. A **spleen scan** using tagged heat damaged RBCs on a patient with fibrosis of the spleen would be expected to show increased hepatic sequestration of cells.
51. To do a **placental scan** with ^{99m}Tc serum albumin, the I.V. dose immediately before scanning in 1 millicurie (mci).
52. The **most frequent site of bone metastases at autopsy** of cancer patients in vertebrae.
53. In doing a BONE SCAN with ^{85}Sr (Strontium nitrate), 30% of the injected dose deposits is bone.
54. The most accurate method for determination of enteric protein loss is **albumin ^{Cr}51 test**.
55. During radioisotope **cisternography** using labelled albumin, the albumin normally passes

through the tentorial incisura and can be observed in the Sylvain fissures at 3 to 4 hours time period.

56. Using ^{99m}Tc for a **brain scanning** agent, suspicious areas on the scan may be caused by those vessels include–
    - Superior frontal veins.
    - Superior anastomotic veins.
    - Superficial middle cerebral veins.
    - Middle meningeal veins.
57. The "DOUGHNUT SIGN" seen on a **brain scan** usually suggests—
    - Glioblastoma.
    - Metastases.
    - Abscess.
58. The "CRESCENT SIGN" seen on a **brain scan** commonly indicates a subdural haematoma.

> ***Note:*** *It can also be seen in pachymeningitis and dural metastases.*

59. After intravenous injection of the pertechnetate solution, ^{99m}Tc is concentrated in – stomach and colon.

> ***Note:*** *It is also concentrated in urinary bladder, mucous and salivary glands, thyroid gland.*

60. When an oral dose of vitamin B_{12} of 0.1 to 0.5 μcg is given to a normal patient the amount absorbed is equal to 70%.
61. During a "SCHILLING TEST" 1000 mcg of unlabeled vitamin B_{12} is given 1 to 2 hours after the test dose to promote renal excretion of absorbed labeled vitamin B_{12}.
62. The dose of radioactive phosphorus necessary to induce a **remission in polycythaemia** is in the order of 7 millicuries (mci).
63. In **red cell volume** studies, false high results are due to–the entire dose not being injected into a vein.
64. **Regarding radioimmunoassay method (RIA)**–

> ***Note:** RIA was 1st described by Yallow and Berson (1959) for serum insulin assay. But it was 1st used by Ekins (1960).*

Broadly RIA has two major uses in medicine.

A. Assessment/Assay of substances (hormonal and others).

B. Clinical application.

A. Assessment/Assay of substances (hormonal and others).

i. *Hormonal Assay*
- Hypothalamic–T_{RF}.
- Anterior pituitary–ACTH, FSH, LH, GH, TSH, α and β MSH.
- Thyroid–T_3, T_4 calcitonin.
- Parathyroid–Parathormone.
- Adrenal cortex–Cortisone, aldosterone.
- Sex hormones–oestrogen, progesterone and testosterone.
- Pancreas–Proinsulin, insulin, glucagon.
- Posterior pituitary–Vasopressin, oxytocin.
- Placenta-hCG.

ii. *Hormone-like substance*
- Angiotensin.
- Bradykinin.
- Brain peptides (opoid peptides)-endorphins.

iii. *Drugs*
- Digoxin.
- Digitoxin.
- Morphine.
- Gentamicin.
- Kanamycin.

iv. *Ferroprotein*
- Ferritin.

v. *Vitamin*
- Vitamin B_{12} (cyancobalamin).
- Folic acid.

vi. *Immunological*
- Anti-haemophilic factor.

- Rheumatoid factor.
- Hepatitis 'B' antigen (Australia antigen).
- Carcinoembryonic antigen (CEA).
- IgE.

Clinical application of RIA

i. Diagnosis, e.g. selection of treatment and follow-up, e.g. **male infertility**-measuring semun FSH, LH and testosterone.

e.g. **Diagnosis of hypothyroidism** - Measurement of TSH level has become an important tool in the diagnosis of hypothyroidism distinguishing between hypothyroidism of thyroid origin and pituitary or hypothalamic hypothyroidism.

e.g. **parathyroid hyperfunction** helps to find out the cause of hypercalcemia.

e.g. **Immunological** - to detect rheumatoid factor, Hepatitis 'B' antibodies and rubella antibodies, etc.

e.g. **Management of hypertension** - to evaluate the renin activity, angiotensin and aldosterone levels are assayed.

ii. *Oncology- Tumour Marker*

Certain tumours eleborated some hormones, proteins or some antigen called as specific TUMOUR MARKERS.

As for example–α-**fetoprotein** to detect liver or testes cancers.

iii. *Therapeutic Drug Monitoring*

RIA helps to adjust drug doses, measurement of drug levels in serum to detect toxicity, e.g. digoxin while the patient is on therapy.

iv. *Research Purposes*

- Sympathomimetics and bronchial asthma.
- Radiolabelled adrenergic receptor antagonists have been used as ligand to study the properties of adrenergic receptors.

- RIA studies has been used in basic research on cell physiology.

- **Organ Scan**

  e.g. Liver scan– ^{99m}Tc tagged to phytate.
  BULIDA tagged with Tc.

> ***Note: Radionuclide scan (RNS) vs. Ultrasound (US)***

- US is quicker and easier than RNS. It can used to visual monitoring during surgery, etc. while RNS is not used for such purpose. Gas in the abdomen does not interfere with the US procedure.

- **Bone Scan (BS)**

  BS depend upon the following factors.
  - increased vascularity.
  - increased osteoblastic activity.
  - increased new collagen deposition.
  - **Some clinical observations like–**
    - Stress fracture.
    - Avascular necrosis of femoral head.
    - Bone metastasis.
    - Bone tumours and arthritis.
    - Breast C_A with pain chest.
    - Arthritis.

  e.g. **Brain scan**–uses ^{99m}Tc per technetate. It can diagnose–
  - Tuberculoma.
  - Brain infarct.
  - Brain abscess.
  - Brain neoplasm.
  - Vascular malformation.
  - Extracerebral haematomas.

> ***Note: Radionuclide scan (RNS) vs. CAT scan.***

Although CAT scan is for superior than RNS still RNS is used in following circumstances with precision.

e.g. **Renal imaging** for varieties of clinical conditions.

e.g. **Renal clearance studies.**
e.g. **Cardiac imaging** - Thallium 201. Tc 99m stannous pyrophosphate imaging.
MUGA studies for ventricular functions.

- **Positron emission tomography (PET)**– As the name indicates PET is an ideal scanning technique which utilizes POSITRON emitting radioisotopes.

> ***Note:*** *This PET technique provides valuable information about regional tissue biochemistry, physiology and pharmacology.*

- PET supplies useful information regarding *in vivo* quantitative measurement of:
  i. Regional blood flow.
  ii. Glucose utilization.
  iii. Oxygen utilization.
  iv. Incorporation of selected amino acids in tissues.

> ***Note:*** *SPECT (Single Photon Emission Computed Tomography) is a recently adopted technique for studying coronary artery disease.*

- **LASER in medicine**
  - Based on the Einstein's principle (1917) and methodology Theodore Maiman (1960) developed the 1st working LASER.

  > ***Note:*** *Subsequently, Bell laboratory (1961) built 1st model.*

  - Types of lasers used in medicine include-- Argon, Argon/Krypton, Tunable Dye and Yttrium-Aluminium-Garnet (YAG).
  - Laser beam is applied in biology and medicine for diagnostic, therapeutic and surgery.
- **Nuclear medicine for therapy**
  - β-(beta) rays have the property to ionize and destroy the tissue close to their sources. This property is being utilized in the **therapeutic nuclear medicine.**

- γ-(gamma) rays cannot cause any internal radiation injury and can be detected externally due to this property it is being used in **diagnostic nuclear medicine.**
- **Lawrence (1933)** used ^{32}P for treating leukaemia.
- **Hertz and Roberts (1942)** used radioiodine for treatment of **Graves' disease**.

- **Nuclear medicine therapy is utilized in following states**:
  i. Polycythaemia rubra vera-P^{32}.
  ii. Bone metastasis in C_A breast or C_A prostate-^{32}P.
  iii. Hyperthyroidism-I^{131}.
  iv. Thyroid cancer-I^{131}.
  v. Malignant Pleural effusion
     a. ^{198}Au or colloidal gold.
     b. ^{32}P-colloidal chromic phosphate.
  vi. Malignant ascites.
  vii. Rheumatoid arthritis-^{198}Au, ^{90}Yr, ^{32}P, ^{169}Er.

12

Radiologic Technology

You Should Know

1. A line drawn between the pupils of the eye is called **interpupillary line**.
2. Rhese position, Camp-Gianturco position, Alexander's position, Pfeiffer position, visualize the → **optic foramen**.
3. **Mayer's position** for the par petrosa requires the skull rotated 45° towards the film and the tube angled 45° towards the feet.
4. **Stenver's projection** specifically visualizes the PETROUS PYRAMIDS.
5. In order to demonstrate both petrous ridges, the occipital bone, the foramen magnum and the dorsum sella, the view must be used is 30° **Towne's view**.
6. In the submento-vertex view of the skull, the planes or lines perpendicular to the film includes–
   - Median plane.
   - Sagittal plane.
   - Coronal plane.

> **Note:** *In the submento-vertex view of the skull the planes or lines not perpendicular to the film is → INTER-ORBITAL line.*

7. The FORAMEN OVALE is best seen in **submento-vertical views** of the skull.
8. The **Glabello-Meatal line** connects the auricular point with the glabella.
9. The **orbito-meatal line** connects the auricular point with the nasion.

10. The TOWNE'S view of the skull is also known as → **Grasby's view**.
11. The correct angulation of the central ray for the **Towne's view** of the skull is 40° to 45° AP.
12. The **foramen magnum** and **jugular foramina** are best demonstrated in the Grasby position at 50° to 60° angulation A-P.
13. In the **Water's position for the maxillary sinuses,** the radiographic baseline forms 37° angle with the plane of the film.
14. The **Caldwell position** has the central ray angled 23° to feet.
15. The "LAW POSITION" is used to study an examination of the **mastoid air cells**.
16. In the **true law position**, the central ray is directed 15° toward the feet - 15° towards the face.
17. The **infraorbito-meatal line** connects the auricular point with the infraorbital margin.
18. The AURICULAR POINT is found at the **external auditory meatus**.
19. The interorbital line is perpendicular to the film in **lateral view**.
20. The **Haas' projection** is the reverse of GRASBY or TOWNE'S antero-posterior projection and produces a comparable results.
21. The SCHULLER PROJECTION is primarily taken to demonstrate the **base of the skull**.
22. In the **Schuller projection**, the infraorbito-meatal line must be to the parallel plane of the film.
23. SINUSES (Paranasal) are photographed in the upright position to demonstrate fluid levels.
24. The criteria for attaining satisfactory radiographic quality would be all image densities translucent.
25. The criteria for attaining satisfactory radiographic quality would be the best overall radiographic density.
26. The criteria for attaining satisfactory radiographic quality would be image detail should not be obscured by fog.

27. A criteria for attaing satisfactory radiographic quality would be like that the contrast should be such that differentiation between densities or details can be readily made.
28. A criteria for attaining statisfactory radiographic quality would be maximum sharpness and true shape of the image.
29. A criteria for attaining satisfactory radiographic quality would be that the part examined should be fully penetrated.
30. A criteria for viewing satisfactory radiographic quality would be proper and adequate illumination.
31. In radiographic quality, the letters "PE" stands for **photographic effect**.
32. In radiographic quality, contrast is directly controlled by **Kilovolts peak**.
33. In radiographic quality, densities are directly controlled by milliampere second and target film distance.
34. In radiographic quality, one of our greatest problems is considered to be fog.
35. The type of radiation called primary is that which emerges from the tube and reaches the patient.
36. A type of radiation that is called secondary or scattered would be that which scatters on contact with the patient.
37. The type of radiation that is called remnant would be that which emerges from the patient and reaches the film.
38. In radiography, the latent image is known as the ionized image in the X-ray film emulsion prior to processing.
39. "Radiographic density" is known as overall blackening of the film.
40. A means of further understanding of radiographic density would be quantity of radiation.
41. A definition of radiographic contrast would be the probable relationship between one density and another.

42. A means of further understanding radiographic contrast would be quality of radiation.
43. **"Short scale contrast"** is defined by more contrast.
44. **"Long scale contrast"** is defined as less contrast.
45. The term **"Direct exposure"** would indicate an exposure without the benefit of intensifying screens.
46. The factors directly affecting radiographic density would be—
    - Milliamperage.
    - Time.
    - Distance.
47. In the projection of the knee to show the intercondyloid fossa. The central ray is directed at right angles to the long axis of the tibia.
48. The "CHASARD-LAPINE" position is a special view for a semi-axial view of the pelvis.
49. The "SELLA TURCICA" is best seen in lateral skull projections.
50. The **"Gaynor Hart"** position is used to demonstrate **carpal canal.**
51. **Lymphography** is most commonly employed for Hodgkin's disease or lymphoma.
52. The **Tunnel** or **intercondylar knee view** is recommended with LOOSE bodies.
53. The antero-posterior oblique view of the cervical vertebra is most frequently used to demonstrate the foramina on the side farther away from the film.
54. The effective focal spot on an X-ray tube appears to be square.
55. The factor that does not determine tube capacity is focal film distance.
56. As a result of Heel effect, the intensity of the X-ray beam is greater toward the cathode side of the beam.
57. An increase in anode speed from 3600 RPM to 10,000 RPM results in increase in short exposure ratings.

58. To decrease the thickness of cut in a tomographic study, we increase tube amplitude.
59. To decrease magnification, we use increase target film distance.
60. To increase detail sharpness, we can increase focal film distance.
61. Poor screen contact reduces definition.
62. The use of a cone results in films of higher contrast.
63. Free electrons are made available in the X-ray tube by thermionic emission.
64. Rotating ANODE is not necessary to produce X-ray radiation in the X-ray tube.
65. The use of filters results in beam of greater intensity.
66. Adding filtration to the X-ray beam results in film with less contrast.
67. The image differs from the latent image in that the latter:
    - Demonstrates reciprocity.
    - Is not affected by heat.
    - Requires development.
68. The **film base** commonly used during the years 1900 until 1924 was **cellulose nitrate**.
69. High contrast in a film may be considered as extended contrast.
70. **Filters** are used to reduce amount of radiation to patient.
71. If we wish to double the density of a given film we can double the **MA factor**.
72. To alter the density of a film but not change its contrast scale we may elect to change M.A.
73. Screen film type most often used in a radiology department is more sensitive to BLUE LIGHT.
74. To obtain a sharpest detail in a film, direct exposure technique is used.
75. GRID RATIO refers to height of lead strips vs. the distance between the lead strips.
76. Two physical factors determine the efficiency of a grid is grid ratio and the number of lead strips per inch.

77. The most important advantages of 3 phase X-ray generation is higher tube ratings for very short exposure times.
78. The use of high Kilovoltage results in films with long scale contrast.
79. A change in MAS results in a direct change of density.
80. When the HI-voltage to X-rays tube is increased penetrating characteristic of the beam changes.
81. The smaller the effective focal spot size the less penumbra.
82. To increase detail sharpness, we should decrease OFD.
83. Electrons moving in X-ray tube are referred to as **cathode rays**.
84. When fast moving electrons are suddenly stopped X-rays are produced.
85. **Heat units** (H.U.) are a product of KVP × MA × time.
86. The use of a grid results in reduction in secondary radiation and an improvement in contrast and definition.
87. The use of intensifying screens results in a decrease in exposure by a factor of atleast 20 times less radiation.

13

General and Regional Radiography

You Should Know

1. The **primary X-ray beam** is most accurately limited with **light beam diaphragm**.
2. **Tissues that are particularly susceptible to radiation** include:
   - Foetus.
   - Bone marrow.
   - Gonads.
3. Regarding **radionuclides used for scintigraphy**:
   - It must emit gamma (g) radiation.
   - It must have a suitable physical half-life.
   - It must have short biological life.
   - It should not be toxic.
4. ^{131}**I-orthoiodohippurate** is used for **kidneys scintigraphy**.
5. **67-gallium citrate** is used for **tumour scintigraphy**.
6. For **pancreatic scintigraphy 75-selenium methionine** is used.
7. The highest **gonad doses** to men are received in the examination of hip including **upper femur**.
8. Regarding **fluoroscopy**:
   - Adequate dark adaptation is essential before fluoroscopy.
   - Lead apron with lead equivalent to 5 mm should be used.
   - Fluoroscopy should never be done if the same information can be got by radiography.
   - High doses are involved.

9. To obtain the **maximum sharpness of image**:
   - Geometrical blur should be minimal.
   - Movement blur should be minimal.
   - Photographic blur should be minimal.
10. To **increase the voltage from 70 to 100 kv** the additional filter of aluminium to the diagnostic tube should give total filtration of 2 mm aluminium.
11. The **use of additional filtration** in mammography is a disadvantage.
12. It is true regarding **reduction in field size** that it–
    - Reduces exposure to the patient.
    - Should always be preferred.
    - Improve the contrast in radiograph.
    - Decreases the scattered radiation.
13. It is true regarding the **effects of the increasing focal film distance** that it–
    - Decreases magnification.
    - Reduces geometrical blur.
    - Increases the required exposure factor.
    - Reduces skin dose to the patient.
14. The **standard optimum distance** used for each radiographic examination with few exception is **90 to 100 cm**.
15. Recognized use of **fast screen** allows:
    - Reduction of mA.
    - Reduction of exposure time.
    - Reduction of Kv.
    - Use of fine focus.
16. For the **examination of particular portion of body,** the exposure factors depend upon:
    - The general body built of the subject.
    - Part of the body to be examined.
    - The structure of the body to be demonstrated.
17. **If a limb is under plaster of Paris** the exposure factor required is twice of the normal exposure factor dose.
18. For **hysterosalpingography**, high kilovoltage technique is employed.

19. Regarding **disadvantage of high kilovoltage technique**:
    - Poor contrast of soft tissue structure.
    - Poor contrast in soft tissue structure.
    - Bone details are poorly visualized.
    - Risk of over penetration.
20. Regarding **advantages of high kilovoltage technique:**
    - Scattered radiation is increased.
    - Radiation dose to the patient is decreased.
    - Heating of X-ray tube is reduced.
    - mAs is reduced.
21. **High kilovoltage technique is advantageous in**–
    - Obstetric radiography.
    - Barium meal study.
    - Lumbosacral spine (lateral view).
22. Regarding **soft tissue radiography**–
    - Has high milliamperes (mAs).
    - Has low kilovoltage (Kv).
    - Radiation dose to the patient increases.
    - Part being examined should not be covered with cloth, etc.
23. **Soft tissue radiography** can be useful to demonstrate:
    - Cysticercosis.
    - Calcification in any soft tissues.
    - Low density foreign body in the soft tissue.
    - Larynx, trachea and bony or cartilages in the soft tissues of neck.
    - Mammography.
24. **Multiple radiography technique is useful in**–
    - Multisection radiography.
    - Where both bone and soft tissue details are needed.
    - To demonstrate trachea suprasternally and retrosternally, in latral view.
25. **Stereography demonstrate a three-dimensional image** by two radiographs.
26. **Macroradiography technique** is useful in:
    - Atlanto-axial articulation.

- Orbital phlebography.
- In the diagnosis of early changes of rheumatoid arthritis in hand.
- Dacrocystography.

27. Recognised use of **subtraction radiography** includes–
    - Dacrocystography.
    - To visualize small vessels obscured by bone in angiography.
    - Location of radio-opque foreign body in eye.
28. The most common method of **subtraction radiography** is photography subtraction.
29. **Tomography** is indicated in:
    - To assess the size and depth of underlying pathology or mass.
    - Positional information where right angle view reveals no significant information.
    - When the overlying structures obscure underlying pathology.

> ***Note:*** *In tomography the patient is usually kept still to produce image blur.*

30. Recognized uses of **inclined plain tomography** include:
    - The kidneys.
    - The sternum.
    - The tracheo-bronchial tree.
31. **Hypocyloidal technique of tomography** is better for viewing petrous bones.
32. Recognised **advantage of multisection tomography** includes:
    - Exposure time gets reduced.
    - Lower Kv is used.
    - Radiation dose to the patient is reduced.
    - All layers of film are recorded at the same plane.
33. **Xeroradiography** is useful in—
    - Mammography.
    - Punctate calcification in soft tissue.
    - Localization of non-metalic foreign bodies.
34. **CAT scan** is useful in—
    - To demonstrate tumour in the orbit.

- To detect site of haemorrhage in brain.
- To demonstrate size and position of ventricles in brain.
- To detect tumour in brain.

35. **Regarding radiography of abdomen**–
    - Exposure is usually made in expiration.
    - It must include domes of diaphragm and symphysis pubis.
    - Spleen and liver are best seen in deep inspiration.
    - Low kilovoltage is used.
36. To show **free gas under the dome of diaphragm** in ill patient LATERAL DECUBITUS view is useful.
37. **Fluoroscopy view** is of choice for investigation of movement of domes of diaphragm.
38. To **assess the size and shape of heart,** the useful view is left lateral with barium.
39. To **demonstrate effusion in interlobar fissure** REVERSE LORDOTIC views is most useful.
40. **Baseline of skull** is represented by a line joining the external auditory meatus and outer canthus of eye.
41. In a case of **Head injury** (skull trauma), lateral view is a must.
42. **Pituitary fossa** is better visualized in lateral view.
43. **20° occipitofrontal view** is most commonly used for orbit.
44. To demonstrate **orbital emphysema in black eye** occipito-mental view erect should be taken.
45. **Lateral oblique view** is useful for mastoid air cells.
46. **Occipito-frontal and sub-mento-vertical views** can be used both for mastoid air cells and internal auditory canals.
47. **Internal auditory canals** of the sides are best visualized in occipitofrontal view.

48. To confirm the **presence of fluid in frontal sinus** erect lateral view is useful.
49. For **investigation of the vertebral column** beside simple radiography, tomography, myelography and discography are required.
50. To demonstrate **intervertebral foramina** of cervical spine oblique view is necessary.
51. Posterior oblique view is diagnostic in **spondylolisthesis** of 5th lumbar vertebra.
52. **Scintigraphy** is used to demonstrate tumour in the vertebral column.
53. TOMOGRAPHY is used to demonstrate an **osteolytic lesion** of less than **1 cm** in diameter.
54. **IVP and barium meal** is used to investigate adjacent structure around vertebral column.
55. **Discography** is used to demonstrate herniation of disc.
56. **Myelography** is used to demonstrate any mass encroaching on the spinal canal.
57. **Gallbladder** is best visualized in prone-oblique view.
58. **Postero-anterior view of wrist** with the ulnar deviation is useful for radiography of scaphoid.
59. The **radiological view** more useful to assess the skeletal age of the patient is dorsi-palmer view of hand including wrist joint.
60. **Routine examination of hip** after trauma and for investigation of congenital anomalies anteroposterior view of both hips are undertaken.
61. After **internal fixation** pin must be shown on the film.
62. After surgery involving a single hip, **anteroposterior view** one view only taken.
63. Anteroposterior view (AP view) of only one hip is usually undertaken after **total hip arthroplasty**.
64. **Von Rosen view** is useful in congenital dislocation of hip joints (CDH).
65. **Radiography of knee joint** includes–
    - Basic antero-posterior view.

- Lateral view.
- Oblique view.

66. **Radiography of Patella** includes–
    - Postero-anterior.
    - Lateral.
    - Skylene view.
    - Oblique view.
67. The view most useful to show angle of **femur** in relation to the conditions like **Genu Valgus** or **Genu Varus** is antero-posterior weight bearing.
68. The view most useful to **demonstrate from ligaments of knee joint** is antero-posterior in forced abduction and adduction.
69. The view most useful to show the **osteo-chondritis of tibial lubercle** is lateral view.
70. **Radiography of ankle joint** includes–
    - Anteroprosterior view.
    - Oblique view.
    - Lateral view.
    - AP view in forced eversion and inversion for torn ligament.
71. **Axial view of calcaneum** is used to demonstrate talocalcaneal bar.
72. **Lateral view of calcaneum** is used to demonstrate calcaneal spur.
73. The view demonstrates **torn ligament of knee** is knee joint antero-posterior in forced abduction and adduction.
74. The view ankle joint antero-posterior in forced eversion and inversion demonstrates **torn ligament of ankle**.
75. Regarding radiography of larynx most useful view is **soft tissue lateral view**.
76. To assess the size and shape of heart, the useful views include **left lateral with barium**.
77. To demonstrate **effusion in interlobar fissure** reverse lordotic views is most useful.
78. Radiologically, posterior-oblique view is most useful to demonstrate **lower lobe collapse.**

79. **Small pneumothorax** is best demonstrated by postero-anterior view on expiration.
80. **Penetrated postero-anterior and lateral views** are useful to demonstrate–
    - Paraspinal shadows.
    - Size and calcification in heart.
    - Bases of lungs covered by large breast shadows.
81. **Lateral view of chest** is useful in revealing:
    - To outline effusion.
    - To outline the collapse segment of lung.
    - Pathology obscured by heart or diaphragm.
    - Depressed sternum.
82. Most useful radiological view of larynx is **soft tissue lateral view.**
83. **Radiography of pharynx** is carried out to demonstrate.
    - Presence of foreign body.
    - Tumour.
    - Abscess.
84. Regarding **radiography of heart and lung** fields–
    - Patient stand in front of upright cassette hold.
    - No radio-opaque object should be left in gown or on the chest.
    - Gonads must be protected.
    - Focus film distance is six feet.
85. Regarding **axial view (skylene) of patella**:
    - Patient lie in prone.
    - Flex leg on knee upto 80-85°.
    - Support leg with the help of bandage around ankle and held in his hand.
    - Tube angle 10°-15° between patella and distal end of femur.
86. **Technetium labelled microsphere** is used to scan lungs.
87. **Technetium labelled human serum albumin** is used to demonstrate placenta.
88. **Technetium sulphur colloid** is used to scan liver.

14

Radiotherapy and Radiation Therapy at a Glance

You Should Know

INTRODUCTION

Radiotherapy is a branch of medicine that involves the application of ionizing/particulate radiations in the treatment of disease processes. It includes both X-rays as well as radium induced radiations or from various artificial radium substitutes.

> **Note:** *The major application of radiotherapy is in field of Neoplasia or cancer treatment so definitely the question of dosage is the main concern in delivering such treatment modality to these patients.*

- Dosage does not mean providing a particular rad but it concerns mainly that how much dose is delivered to the patient in how much time and what should be the interval between the two dosages.
- These radiation dosages are measured precisely and accurately by sensitive physical instruments like—
  i. Geiger Muller counter.
  ii. Proportional counters.
  iii. Pocket Dosimeters.
  iv. Film Badges.
  v. Thermo Luminescent dosimeter.

> **Note:** *Most commonly used monitoring badges for personnel monitoring includes–Film Badge and Thermo Luminescent Dosimeter (TLD).*

- Both film Badge and TLD are capable of using absorbed doses from 1 m rad to thousands of rads. However, TLD badges is more accurate and consistent than the film badge.

- **Recognised Advantage of TLD Badges**
  a. Fast reading capabilities during emergency.
  b. Serve as dosimetry system for patient exposure monitoring and making other exposure measurement.
  c. Less likely to give false positive or negative reading due to changes in environmental parameters like heat, light and pressure.
- **Recognised Advantage of Film Badges**
  a. Compared to TLD, it is cheap.
  b. It records exposure permanently so it can be stored for future reference and re-evaluation.
- **Dose Measurement (DM)**

> ***Note:*** *In radiotherapy, accurate DM is absolutely necessary. The purpose of the measurements is to obtain reliable "absorbed dose" information at any point in the patient's body.*

- **Absorbed Dose (AD)**
  It is defined as the amount of energy absorbed from a beam of radiation per unit mass of the absorbing material.
- **Potency of Radiation (POR)**

Note: POR is measured by ***Roentgen, Rad and Rem****.*

i. **Roentgen** is the unit of exposure as a measure of the radiation being delivered to a particular area.

> ***Note:*** *The amount of ionisation by a beam of radiation in air is measured and this is called* ***"Radiation Exposure"****.*

- **Roentgen** is defined as "the amount of radiation absorbed in air at a given point i.e. number of ions produced in 1 (one) ml of air".

  Currently Roentgen is replaced by S1 units like coulomb/kg.

  One Roentgen = 2.58 × 10 coulomb/kg air.

> ***Note:*** *The Roentgen is limited to X-rays and γ-rays upto 3 MV (million volt).*

ii. **Rad** is the most commonly used unit of radiation dose. It is the unit of "absorbed dose". Because the energy actually transferred to irradiated volume is responsible for causing biological changes, so "Rad" is the amount of radioactive energy absorbed per gram of tissue or any material.

Currently "Rad" is replaced by Gray (Gy).

Gray (Gy) = 1 Joule/kg or 1 Gray = 100 rads.

> ***Note:*** *For each Rad delivered, each gram of tissue will absorb an energy of 100 ergs.*

iii. **Rem** is the product of absorbed dose and the modifying factors. In fact, it indicates the degree of potential dangers to health.

> ***Note:*** *Current concept is that Maximum Permissible Dose (MPD) should not be **> 5 rems** over a period of 30 years to entire population from all communities/societies.*

QUANTITY OF RADIOACTIVITY (QOR)

- **Curie** is the amount of radon in equilibrium with one gram of radium. Since, newer radioisotopes have been introduced into the clinical practice, so a new unit of quantity of radioactivity should be introduced. In its new form curie is not the unit of quantity but a unit of activity. So, it is defined as number of disintegrations per second.

Therefore, 1 curie = 3.7×10^{10} disintegrations per second.

or 1 curie = 3.7×10^{10} Becquerel (Bq).

CONCEPT OF IONISING RADIATIONS (IR)

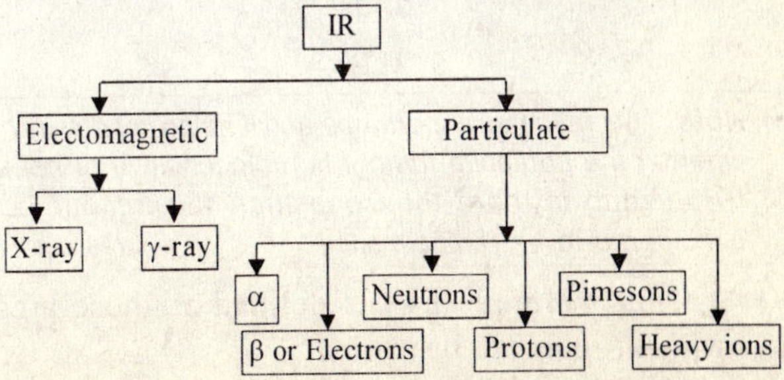

- The properties of X-rays and γ-rays are same. The only difference in between them is that X-rays are produced by X-ray tube as artificial production while γ-rays are produced by radioactive substances which can be natural like Radium, Thorium etc. and artificial like cobalt 60 and Caesium 137 etc.

What is Half Value Layer (HVL)?

Definition

The thickness of absorber needed to reduce or cut down the dose by one half is called HVL. It is expressed in mm or cm.

It is a method of measuring radiation quality (type of radiation).

Quality is changed by filteration. An increase in either atomic number or the thickness of the filter increase the penetrating ability of the beam. In other words half value layer (HVL) increases. Above 1 mm Cu, an increase of HVL decreases the back scatter factor because an increasingly greater percentage of radiation is scattered in forward direction and less in lateral or backward direction.

> ***Note:*** *The material used for HVL includes copper (Cu), Lead (Pb) or Aluminium (Al) etc.*

What is Tumour Lethal Dose (TLD)?

TLD is defined as the dose which is lethal to the tumour as a whole, killing the tumour completely and it provides complete and permanent regression of the tumour mass.

What do you mean by Therapeutic Ratio (TR)?

TR is the ratio of NTT (Normal Tissue Tolerance) to the TLD. It is expressed as

$$\frac{\text{NTT}}{\text{TLD}}$$

> ***Note:*** *This ratio has importance and it helps in knowing whether the particular tumour is radiosensitive or not. If the ratio is more than one then the tumour is considered to be radiosensitive.*

- **Target Volume (TV)** is defined as those area which is going to be treated.

- **Tumour volume** is defined as the gross tumour area plus its microscopic extension which cannot be seen with naked eye.
- **Tumour Dose (TD)** is defined as the dose which goes maximum in a block of tissue, or it is the absorbed dose in rads at a particular location of the tumour.
- **Modal Dose (MD)** is defined as the dose which is occurring most frequently at different points in whole block of tissue.
- **Percentage Depth Dose (PDD)**–At a given point, it is the ratio (expressed as percentage) of the absorbed dose at that point to the absorbed dose at the dosage reference point.

$$PDD = \frac{\text{Absorbed dose at the point}}{\text{Absorbed dose at surface}} \times 100$$

FACTORS INFLUENCING PERCENTAGE DEPTH DOSE

a. **Depth of tumour** is the most important factor which affects PDD. As the depth of the tumour increases the dose rate decreased because of the attenuation of the beam through absorption, scattering and inverse square law.

b. **Dimension of the field size:** As the area of the field increases, there is a corresponding increase in the volume of the irradiated tissue with resulting increase in the % of scattered radiation. The scattered radiations are added to primary radiation reaching a given point below the surface and therefore it contributes to an increased percentage depth dose.

> ***Note:*** *PDD is smaller in rectangular field than square field.*

c. **Skin to Source Distance (SSD):** Owing to less divergence of the rays at the greater SSD, a large fraction of the surface exposure rate reaches a given depth below the surface.

So, more the SSD, greater is the percentage depth dose.

MODE OF ADMINISTRATION OF RADIOTHERAPY

> ***Note:*** *Radiotherapy can be delivered to human by either Brachytherapy or Teletherapy.*

Brachytherapy means treating the tumour with radiation sources that are inserted into the tumour or are kept very near to the tumour.

i. If they are kept into the tumour it is called INTERSTITIAL therapy like cheek, tongue etc.
ii. When they are kept inside the body then it is called INTRACAVITARY brachytherapy. As for example–Uterus, Vagina, Esophagus etc.

Advantages of Brachytherapy

a. It delivers a particular dose in a very short time.
b. The sources remain in contact with tumour and tissues continuously.
c. It spares the nearby normal tissue.
d. It can effectively control dose distribution.

Disadvantages of Brachytherapy

a. Needs admission in hospital ward.
b. The reaction of radiations does not allow to be checked.
c. Dose calculations at the tumour volume and normal areas has to be very exact and accurate.
d. Difficulty in applying in inaccessible sites.
e. Very few patients may be treated at a given tissue.

Teletherapy means treating the tumour by radiations that are kept at a distance like X-ray machine, cobalt^{60} therapy etc.

Advantages of Teletherapy

a. More patients in number may be treated daily.

b. Radiation reaction may be checked and monitored regularly.
c. It offers radiation administrations in inaccessible sites.
d. Dose distribution to the area given in respect of anatomy may be better controlled owing to its various field sizes and diaphragms.

Disadvantages of Teletherapy

a. Patient has to come daily for few weeks for radiotherapy.
b. Surrounding normal tissue also gets radiation exposure.

GAMMA (γ) RADIATIONS

> **Note:** *γ radiations has to be delivered to treat the patients problems by means of two processes like kilovoltage and megavoltage radiations.*

- **Kilovoltage Radiations** are the radiations having energy < 1 million electron volt (< MeV).
- **Megavoltage Radiations** are the radiations having energy more than > 1 million electron volt (> MeV).

DIFFERENCE BETWEEN KILOVOLTAGE RADIATIONS AND MEGAVOLTAGE RADIATIONS

a. **Megavoltage has better penetrating power,** so produce a better depth dose.
   As for example–For a field of 10×10 cm^2 at 10 cm depth the percentage depth dose as follows:
   - Kilovoltage radiations 35%
   - 4 MeV 60%
   - 20 MeV 80%

> **Note:** *This means the higher the voltage the better is the penetration.*

b. Since there is better penetration with megavoltage radiation and less skin dose, the **treatment can be delivered by less number of fields.** This helps in planning the treatment schedule.

c. **Megavoltage has the advantage of skin sparing effect.** This is due to maximum build up below skin depending upon the energy used, which can be summarised as follows:

• 4 MeV	20%
• 20 MeV	12%
• Cobalt	25%
• Kilovoltage	100%

> ***Note:*** *From the above it is clear that in Megavoltage radiation there are less skin reactions whereas in kilovoltage radiations one sees very severe skin reactions of almost cent percent.*

d. **Megavoltage radiations offers the advantage of bone sparing effect.** This is due to the fact that in kilovoltage radiation there is photoelectric absorption of radiations, therefore the tumour getting lesser dose whereas in megavoltage radiation range there is no photoelectric absorption effect.

Brachytherapy uses the following Radioisotopes

i. Ra226 – Radium.
ii. Cs137 – Caesium.
iii. Co60 – Cobalt.
iv. Ir192 – Iridium.

Teletherapy uses the following Radioisotopes

i. Cobalt ii. Caesium.

Recognised characteristics of various radioisotopes most commonly used in present day clinical practice of Radiotherapy.

i. **Radium** – Ra226 used for Brachytherapy purposes.

– Energy	0.19–2.43 MeV
– Half life	1620 years
– Rate of decay (approx.)	1% per 25 years
– K factor	(R/h-mci at 1 cm) 8.25.

> ***Note:*** *Now-a-days it has been not used clinically but it needs mention in radiotherapy.*

Advantages of Radium

- It has a constant dose rate.
- Most of the calculations are based on Radium.
- It has a very-very long half life.

Disadvantages of Radium

- It has potentiality to release radioactive RADON GAS which may leak out owing to defective instruments or careless procedure.
- Low specific activity of approx. 1 curie per gram, so the size of source will be bigger.
- Very high photon energy make the protection of the source housing difficult.
- Because it emits all types of radiations like (α, β and γ rays) and if α particles gets absorbed and would remain active during a very long physical and biological half life.

ii. **Caesium (Cs137)**

> ***Note:*** *It can be used in both Brachytherapy as well as Teletherapy.*

- Now-a-days it is used mainly as Brachytherapy because it has a low specific activity plus low K factor. Caesium units operate at source skin distance of < 40 cm and thus the beam has a wide pneumbra (focus) and there are severe skin reactions when used in teletherapy.

Characteristics of Caesium

• Energy	0.662 MeV.
• Half life	30 years.
• Rate of Decay	1% per 6 months, 2% per annum or year so source can be replaced after 20 years.
• K factor	(R/h-mci at 1 cm)—3.3.
• Typical SSD	20 to 40 cm.

> ***Note:*** *For Teletherapy purposes the energy is lower and for Brachytherapy purposes it is ideal, though little higher, so necessary protection is comparatively cheaper and higher.*

- It has an advantage that it can reproduce the dosimetry of radium which was used previously and to which Radiotherapist is accustomed and well acquainted.

iii. **Cobalt (Co60)**

> ***Note:*** *Co 60 is used for both Brachy as well as Teletherapy purposes.*

- The effective photon energy of Co 60 is only slightly lower than that of radium and its half life is relatively short making it a choice isotope to be used in Teletherapy unit.
- It can be made to a high specific activity which combined with K factor of 13R/m-mci at 1 cm produce a source with a high useful beam exposure rate.

> ***Note:*** *Owing to its short half life, treatment time have to be increased by approx. 1% per month.*

Characteristics of Cobalt 60

Energy-γ ray	1.17 MeV, 1.33 MeV (average 1.25 MeV).
Half life	5.3 years so in practice have to be replaced once every 3 to 4 years interval.
Rate of decay	1% per month.
K-factor	(R/-mci at 1 cm) 13.0.

RADIOTHERAPY TREATMENT PLANNING (RTP)

Introduction

The **aim** of proper RTP is to deliver homogenous dose of radiation to "tumour volume" with minimal or possibly negligible effect on nearby or adjacent normal tissues.

> ***Note:*** *Basically the RTP means the work involved in displaying graphically a dose distribution which results when one or more radiation beams converge on the treatment volume.*

WHAT IS TREATMENT VOLUME AND TREATED VOLUME?

i. **Treatment Volume** is defined as follows by the clinician as being the tumour or lesions surrounded by margins he/she chooses to include in the treatment.

ii. **Treated Volume** is defined as that volume which is actually covered by radiation beams and raised to a prescribed level of dose.

Criteria for Optimum Treatment Plan

a. The dose throughout the treatment volume should be uniform to within ± 5% of tumour dose.

b. The treated volume should be as near as possible be the same as treatment volume in position, size and shape.

c. The dose to the treated volume should exceed that to any area by atleast say 20%.

d. The dose to neighbouring radiosensitive sites (e.g. eye, spinal cord etc.) should, where practicable, be kept below the tolerance dose.

e. The integral dose should be kept to minimum. Integral dose is the summation of the dose to all elements of irradiated tissue and represents the total energy absorbed.

Distribution of Radiation

Types of Field Choosen

i. Parallel pair
   - Parallel and opposed pair.
   - Mid point receives the minimum dose along the central axes and maximum dose at right angles to the central axes.

- Within limits—the tissue irradiated receives a uniform dose and variation of dose is increased if the separation is more or energy is less.
- Technique is valuable where large volumes of tissues are irradiated or where the treatment is palliative.

BOX TECHNIQUE

If parallel pair gives uniform irradiation to the enclosed tissues, then two intersecting parallel pairs will produce even distribution over the volume enclosed by all the four fields. The distribution is "square" when two pairs are at right angles or they may produce a "diamond" distribution when two pairs are say at 120 degree.

The disadvantage of this technique is that when small fields are used at large separations, the irradiated tissue outside the treated volume receives half the dose to that inside. This may lead to dose exceeding the tolerance level of critical structures like spinal cord.

As for example: C_A C_X, C_A Urinary bladder, C_A Prostate etc.

THREE FIELD TECHNIQUES

Here the arrangement of the fields are such that they only overlap in the treated volume thereby reducing the dose to the critical organs to the minimum.

As for examples–C_A bronchus, C_A Esophagus.

BEAM MODIFICATIONS

The effect of beam radiation may be modified by using a tissue compensator or wedge.

> ***Note:*** *Combinations of two or three fields are used most commonly.*

Tissue compensator is placed in the beam path to correct dose in homogenicity due to varying depth of tumour volume or obliquity or contour.

The **charted isodose curve** may be used while maintaining the skin sparing properties of the mega-voltage beam by the use of tissue compensators. Here the lack of attenuation in the region of tissue deficiency is made good by using an attenuator in the beam sufficiently removed from the skin that the built up region is unaffected.

> ***Note:*** *This technique is very useful in areas where skin curvature is complex e.g. in Head and Neck tumours.*

Wedge filters: When the tumour is placed eccentrically or where the treatment volume is close to the surface of the patient but too thick to be adequately treated by a single field, it is often convenient to use two beams with wedges. Basically the wedge helps in producing a satisfactory dose distribution where fields overlap.Therefore, it avoids high dose area and low dose areas in areas of field overlapping. This is very useful in treatment of regions like maxillary antrum, larynx, middle ear, eye and urinary bladder.

> ***Note:*** *Wedge filter techniques are of great value at megavoltage radiation levels than at kilovoltage levels. This wedge can be made of any metal.*

The wedge is more often positioned in beam immediately behind the minor of the light beam diaphragm. The basic purpose of the use of the wedge is that it attenuates the beam on one side of the beam axis relative to the other, thereby tilting the isodose curve through an angle.

Wedge angle is the angle through which 50% isodose line is turned.

Ideal dose distribution using wedge is achieved when two beams of wedge angle are used with a hinge angle of (180-20°) degrees, where the hinge angle is the angle between the beam axes at their point of intersection. Wedge fields are always used in pairs with their thick ends together.

Role of Immobilization helps to maintain the treatment position accurately thereby enhancing the accuracy of the treatment planning. This is usually done by **Perspex Shell** or **Cast**. This ensures the reproducibility so that the treatment volume remains the same during the entire treatment otherwise some areas will get more dose while others will get less dose.

Tumour localization: Treatment of megavoltage radiation planned using a "simulator". It simulates the treatment conditions, means it has all the features of radiotherapy machine like **Couch, Gantry, Collimated wires** etc. but has X-ray tube.

The distance of source of radiation to skin is set to correspond to that of a specific treatment machine and the field is defined by moving the position of cross wires in simulator to correspond to treatment volume required. The X-ray film is taken and the areas are well confirmed which will simulate when the treatment is done by the radiotherapy machine.

Beam direction devices are those enabling the beam axis to be directed at the lesion in the planned direction at a predetermined point and distance from the source of radiation.

> ***Note:*** *The widely used beam directed devices are front and back points, pin and arc isocentric gantry.*

A BRIEF INTRODUCTION TO TUMOUR OR NEOPLASIA OR MALIGNANCY

Definition of Neoplasia: It means abnormal growth but it was R.L. Willis who probably defined in a best way like "Abnormal mass of tissue, growth of which is excessive and incoordinated and persists in the same fashion even after the cessation of the stimulus that evokes the changes".

Neoplasia can be **Benign** or **Malignant**.

Recognised Presentation of Malignancy

- Lump or sore or ulcer.
- Change in bladder or bowel habits.
- Abnormal menstrual bleeding.
- Change in voice or persistent cough.
- Difficulty in eating/breathing.
- Blood in urine/stool/or sputum.
- Persistent fever/loss of weight/loss of appetite.
- Intractable pain.

Recognised Modes of Spread of Tumour

- Local spread.
- Spread by lymph nodes.
- Spread by blood stream.
- Spread through cavity.

Local spread ensues owing to too rapid proliferation of malignant cells resulting in formation of a mass. This may cause ulceration, may cause bleeding or secondary infections. This may lead to pressure changes in form of obstruction (e.g. in Esophagus, lungs, may effect brain leading to headache or convulsions) or may erode a blood vessel leading to bleeding.

Spread through lymphatics/lymph nodes ensues from primary focus to one or more regional lymph nodes.

As for example – Axillary nodes in C_A breast.
– Pelvic nodes in C_A cervix.

> **Note:** *From one group of nodes the disease may spread to other lymph nodes e.g. from axilla to other axilla in C_A breast and then to supraclavicular nodes.*

Spread by blood stream ensues in malignant cells by direct invasion of capillaries or veins of through lymph vessels.

Carcinoma when spread through blood stream it denotes late stage as seen in C_A lung, C_A liver, renal cell C_A etc.

> **Note:** *Spread by blood mainly seen in sarcomatous growth.*

Spread through Cavity: As for example in C_A ovary cancer cells may spread to peritoneal surfaces.

> **Note:** *In Medulloblastoma whole of CSF is considered to be at risk.*

Staging of cancer is done to define the extent of disease. It helps in deciding about the treatment and prognosis.

> **Note:** *Staging can be done only on the basis of clinical findings or can incorporate pathological findings.*

Most commonly employed system are simplified and TNM classification.

Simplified System of Tumour Staging

- Stage I – Tumour confined to organ of origin.
- Stage II – Local lymph nodes involved.
- Stage III – Distant nodes are involved or local spread of disease beyond organ of origin.
- Stage IV – Blood born metastasis.

TNM Classification of Tumour

This TNM system is proposed for international use to have a uniform method all over the world to express the size and the extent of spread of the disease on which depends its staging its treatment and its prognosis.

T : Stands for local extension of primary tumour.
N : Refers to status of regional nodes.
M : Refers to presence of distant metastasis.

T *is further subdivided into:*

T_1 & T_2 : Growth very small and is confined to organ of origin relatively larger growth.

T_3 & T_4 : Very large growth infiltrating into the neighbouring structures.

N *further subdivided into:*

N_1 : Nodes are mobile and are on the same side of primary disease.

N_2 : Mobile nodes of opposite side.

N_3 : Fixed nodes.

M *further subdivided into:*

M_0 : No evidence of distant metastasis.

M_1 : Distant metastasis present.

PRINCIPLES OF TREATMENT OF ANY TUMOUR

A. General assessment of the patient

a. **General condition of the patient:** Whether good or poor, any associated history of diabetes, hypertension etc.

b. **Define the extent of disease:** The local, regional and distant spread is defined accurately and all the patients are staged accurately.

i. **Clinical examination:** It is of great value in defining the local extent of disease particularly of accessible site like cervix, oral cavity, breast etc. Simultaneously regional nodes can also be assessed in regions like breast, oral cancers.

ii. **Diagnostic tools:** Radiography like X-ray chest for primary or secondaries, in chest, skeletal survey for secondaries in bone, soft tissue neck for head and neck cancers, lymphangiogram for nodes in pelvic and para aortic regions.

These days with the advent of imaging techniques like CAT scan, ultrasound, isotope scan, MRI, etc. tumours can be better delineated at very early stage. Thus the chances of cure or control would increase.

Endoscopies like bronchoscopy for lung, cystoscopy for urinary bladder are very valuable for establishing disease in these regions.

iii. FNAC and cell cytology for fluids.

iv. Histopathology provides the degree of differentiation and its biological behaviour. It also helps in defining the choice of treatment.

B. Radical or Palliative Treatment

- **Radical treatment** is given with an aim to cure the disease. The treatment is directed towards primary as well as its possible areas of spread. For example in C_A oral cavity, along with primary disease nodes of both sides are included in radiation field. In C_A breast along with chest wall, all regional nodes in axilla, supraclavicular region and internal mammary nodes are included in radiation treatment.
- **Palliative treatment** is considered when radical treatment is considered to be impracti-

cal because of age, poor general condition or very advance disease. In this form of treatment, aim is only to relieve the symptoms like pain, bleeding or stalling fungation or pathological fracture thereby improving the quality of rest of patient's life.

- **Modes of treatment of malignancy**
  - Surgery (ST).
  - Radiotherapy (RT).
  - Chemotherapy (CT).
  - Immunotherapy (IT).
  - Hormonal therapy (HT).
- **Surgery or radiotherapy** depends upon various factors like site, operability, radiosensitivity and histopathology.
  - i. **Site**–Some primaries are definitely considered for primary surgery, if they are amenable to total surgical resection like, operable growth of breast, lungs, G.I.T., kidney, brain tumours, malignant melanoma, etc.
  - ii. **Operability**–C_A oesophagus of upper one-third is technically difficult to operate because nearby so many vital mediastinal structures as well as C_A breast if fixed to chest wall is almost inoperable.
  - iii. **Radiosensitivity**
    - a. **Poorly sensitive sarcomas**

> ***Note:*** *It is not only the radiosensitivity that dictates the radiation results but also the extent of disease and potential areas of spread which may limit the high doses to be administered.*

As for example: Both Hodgkin's and medulloblastomas are very sensitivie to radiations but very large fields are to be treated limiting the high doses to be delivered.

b. **Moderately sensitive tumours**
- C_A breast.
- C_A lung.
- C_A skin.
- C_A ovary.
- C_A cervix (C_AC_X).

c. **Highly sensitive tumours**
- Lymphoma–Hodgkin's disease.
- Wilms' tumour.
- Seminoma testis.
- C_A ovary.
- Ewings sarcoma.

Role of Chemotherapy

- It can be used as adjuvant to control micro-metastasis, palliative or may be treatment of choice. Role as adjuvant, e.g. in C_A breast, osteosarcoma, nonseminomatous testicular tumour, as palliative in C_A oral cavity, as the treatment of choice in acute leukaemia, choriocarcinoma, lymphomas.
- Hormones have role in—
  - C_A breast.
  - C_A prostate.
  - Uterine tumours.
  - C_A thyroid.

A BRIEF INTRODUCTION TO RADIOBIOLOGY

A. *Cellular response to Radiation*

> **Note:** *Usually two types of effects are observed following radiation.*

- Loss of normal functioning of the cell means cell stops functioning.
- Loss of ability for reproduction means cells cannot multiply.

B. *Cell cycle includes $G_1 \rightarrow S \rightarrow G_2 \rightarrow M$ phases and G_0 phase.*

- **G_1-phase** : Here replication of RNA ensues, length varies from minutes to years.

> **Note:** *G_1 phase is resistant to Radiotherapy (RT).*

- **S-phase** : Here synthesis or DNA ensues length varies from 6 to 50 hours.

> **Note:** *Most resistant to radiotherapy.*

- **G_2 phase :** Here cell prepares for subsequent mitosis length of phase is less than 6 hours.

> ***Note:*** *Sensitive to radiotherapy.*

- **M-phase :** Here cell divides into two daughter cells by process of mitosis.
  - Lenth of 'M' phase is about one hour.

> ***Note:*** *Cells are most sensitive to radiotherapy.*

- **G_0 phase :** It is resting phase. Here cell is not proliferating but performing other normal specified functions.

> ***Note:*** *This G_0 phase is resistant to* ***radiotherapy.***

C. Cell Survival Curve (CSC)

- CSC curve exhibits the relationship between the dose given and % of irradiated cells surviving with the ability to reproduce.
- Any given dose will kill a certain % of cells. The remaining cells after temporary inhibition of mitosis, will recover and if the same dose is applied again the same % of cells will be killed and so on.
- Cell survival curve has following features—

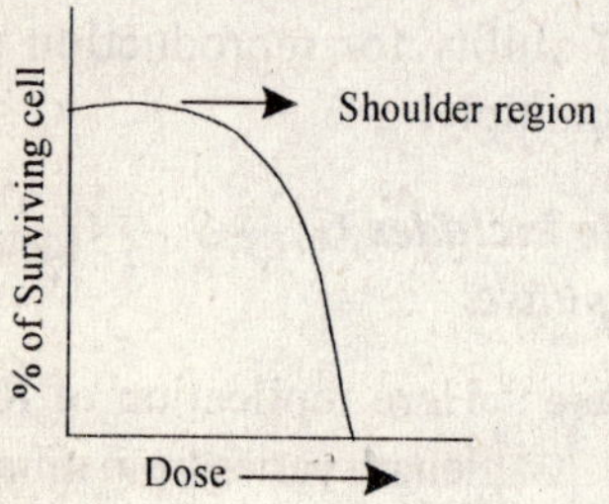

- After moderate dose there is a small shoulder after which the curves become a straight line. The shoulder region is because of sublethal damage and cell recovery, i.e. a proportion of cells recover rapidly in the course of next 4 to 6 hours.

- Since the aim of proper treatment planning is that cancer cells should be killed to the maximum while sparing the normal tissues, therefore, the single dose is fractionated or divided into fractions and total dose is administered over few weeks so that there is time for normal cells to recover. If the total dose is given in a single fraction, of course the cancer cells will die, but simultaneously the normal cells will also not recover.

FACTOR MODIFYING RADIATION EFFECTS

A. O_2

In presence of O_2, radiation causes more cell killing. Therefore, if the blood supply to the irradiated volume is poor or the patient is anaemic, the response to radiation is poor.

B. Dose Rate

Dose/minute : If dose rate is higher, then there will be more cell killing.

C. Quality Factor: RBE and LET

Linear energy transfer (LET) is energy delivery per unit length along the track of radiation. High LET (e.g. a particles, neutrons) means densly ionising, dissipating more energy per unit length of its path than less densly ionising radiations (e.g. γ-rays).

> ***Note:*** *The high LET radiation is more efficient than low.*

This factor is measured by relative biological effectiveness or RBE. This helps in comparing between the biological effects of different qualities of radiation used in clinical practice. It is defined as the ratio of the (absorbed) doses which produce the same biological effects.

Since for historical reasons, the effects of 250 KV, are most familiar so, this energy is used as baseline.

RBE = Absorbed dose for biological effect at 250 KV.

Absorbed dose for same effect at quality in question.

If RBE of 250 KV is 1, then RBE of other energies are:

Cobalt 60 –	80	– 95
	4 MV	– 85
	20 MV	– 80.

FRACTIONATION

Here the total dose is not given in one day or in single sitting. The dose is divided into various fractions, usually 200 rads are given daily.

As for example–if total dose to be given is 6000 rads then it will be delivered in 30 days (200 × 30 = 600).

The advantages of fractionation include:

a. Patient can tolerate radiotherapy in a better way.
b. Better tissue and tumour response.

RADIOBIOLOGY, RADIATION AND ITS EFFECTS ON NORMAL TISSUES

> ***Note:*** *The response to radiation on tissue is being presented by summation of cellular effects on parenchymal cells and vascular stromal cells.*

In tissues having static population, having non-dividing parenchymal cells (e.g., neurons in CNS), following radiotherapy, the critical damage is supposed to occur in vascular compartment, whereas the parenchymal cells of such tissues are relatively radio-resistant.

While in tissues with dividing parenchymal cell, the radiations cause damage of both vascular compartment as well as the parenchymal cell compartment. Therefore, a dose of radiation which kill most of the skin cell of the parenchymal compartment, will subsequently lead to depletion of functioning mature cells. In this kind of system, tissues having shortest turnover times are affected the earliest. Repopulation of stem cells and mature cells by the remaining stem cells play an important part in regaining tissue function after radiotherapy.

> ***Note:*** *The recognised examples in this kind of system are, G.I.T. skin, testis and haemopoietic system.*

Reaction in Normal Tissue

Radiotherapy to a treatment volume by giving radiations more than the limits of tolerance is being accompanied or followed by a reaction in the treated zone. They may manifest in the form of early reactions or late reaction or both. Although unavoidable, every effect should be made to relieve the discomfort by proper and careful nursing.

Reaction of Skin

- In cutis or skin there is a **latent period** of ten days or more depending upon the rate of input of dose before a visible reaction is seen. After this a gradually increasing erythema ensues. This follows the phase of moist desquamation which usually develops approximately at dose of 4500–6000 rads and usually 5 to 6 weeks from start of therapy.
- During **moist desquamation** the superficial layer of the epidermis is shed. The phase of moist desquamation goes on directly to **fibrinous exudation** which may last as long as several weeks.
- During fibrinous exudation the treated area is completely denuded of superficial epidermis,is raw, tender, and if touched bleed easily.
- The reaction subsides through a phase of re-epithelialization usually with much crusting to fading erythema and return to normal when tolerance limits in skin and mucous membrane are exceeded, this may lead to necrosis, where the reaction fails to head and ingested goes on to form an ulcer with sharp edges and is very painful.

> **Note:** *It is to be noted that, although Kilovoltage therapy may not be in regular use having in present day radiotherapy practice, such reactions had often to be accepted inevitable even in the uninvolved skin in the entrance field of beam used for full dosage irradiation of deeper tumours.*

- By judicious use of megavoltage radiations this can be avoided.

  Instructions for care of skin to the patients:

  i. Patient should be told about the reactions as normal accompaniments of reactions. They should be reassured that they will improve gradually in the following weeks.

  ii. Do not apply heat (no hot bath or hot water bottle) or use cold (no ice bags).

  iii. Do not scratch or shave the treated area.

- **Treatment of local reaction** depends on the facts that the less these reactions are interfered with, the better is the healing.

> **Note:** *The ideal treatment is to keep the damaged skin dry as long as possible while avoiding friction.*

- When moist desquamation ensues, it is still advisable to keep the part exposed. For the sake of psychological satisfaction 0.75% gention violet in water is advised to be applied locally.
- **Alopecia** is a problem of radiotherapy when hair bearing area is included in the treated zone.

> **Note:** *ALOPECIA usually begins about three weeks after the start of radiotherapy and progresses rapidly. Epilation ensues at comparatively low dose levels.*

- Regrowth of hair is usually seen 3 months later and nearly full regrowth might be reasonably expected in most patients.

> **Note:** *Changes in hair texture and even colour may be seen. The new hair tend to be finer than the original.*

REACTIONS SEEN IN MUCOSA

After a latent period, an early erythema (often seen rarely) develops rapidly followed 1st by a patchy, later on by a complete whitish yellow membrane covering the entire radiated area. Around this there may be a red-marginal border.

> ***Note:*** *During the course of radiation treatment both skin and mucosal reactions are painful.*

Depending upon the site, patient may have odynophagia, dysphagia, hoarseness in reaction of larynx, dysuria in reaction of the urinary bladder. Xerostomia may also manifest during therapy while treating head and neck cancers. This is a persistent problem. While irradiating abdomen, there may be pseudo-diarrhoea which may necessitate stopping the treatment temporarily.

Delayed reactions largely results from damage to cells that survive but regain some legacy of radiation exposure. Delayed complications that follow radiotherapy usually manifest after months or years. Therefore, it is important to look for these problems at the time of routine follow-up visits and consider the possibility of radiation complications in the differential diagnosis of problems that ensue later in these patients.

> ***Note:*** *Most delayed complications usually appear during the 1st two years period.*

The organ affected depends upon the site of radiotherapy, volume irradiated, daily fraction size, concurrent disease and tolerance of the organ irradiated in the field.

GENETIC (MUTAGENIC) EFFECTS OF RADIATIONS

Radiation may cause mutations. Any dose of radiation, however, small can lead to mutation and chromosomal changes therefore entailing genetic risk.

> **Note:** *It has been seen that the radiation amounting to one rem per 30 examination increases the incidence of mutations by approximately 1%.*

CARCINOGENESIS

There is a definite correlation between radiation exposure and carcinogenesis. The common malignancies where there is a growing evidence that radiation produces C_A thyroid in those who had received radiotherapy treatment to head and neck region several years back and leukaemia in patient treated by total nodal irradiation and chemotherapy.

So, mutagenesis and carcinogenesis are potential hazards not only for patient being treated by radiotherapy but also for persons occupationally exposed to ionising radiations. Present concept point towards ALARA meaning as low as reasonably achievable.

Along with the cancer cells, normal cells are also irradiated. But normal tissues have a strong natural tendency to organise themselves again by normal repair mechanisms, they will be able to regrow. But in cancer, cells have very impaired powers of repair mechanisms.

> **Note:** *A radiotherapist should be alert for any skin reactions and if reactions occur, he must stop the radiotherapy for the time being.*

Regional radiotherapy includes the treatment of several organ system of human with the help of radiotherapy.

CARCINOMA BREAST (C_A BREAST)

Higher Risk Factors

- Positive family history.
- Prior breast cancer.
- Gross cystic disease.
- Prior history of intraductal papilloma.
- Prior history of endometrial C_A.
- Childless women and those conceiving after the age of 30.

Simplified staging of Breast Cancer

Stage I – Disease is confined to breast. Freely movable. There are no suspicious nodes.

Stage II – As above, but axillary node(s) mobile palpable on same side.

Stage III – Primary disease in breast more extensive than stage I, e.g. skin may be invaded, or disease may have fixicity to underlying muscle.
Axillary nodes, if positive are fixed or supraclavicular nodes may be involved.

Stage IV – Extension of disease beyond chest area, e.g. opposite breast may be involved or opposite axilla may have positive nodes or there may be evidence of distant metastasis.

Clinical-TNM Classification

T – Primary tumour
- T1 – Diameter 2 cm or less - not fixed. Includes Paget's disease.
- T2 – Tumour diameter 2 to 5 cm-not fixed.
- T3 – Tumour diameter > 5 cm.
- T4 – Skin or chest wall involvement (Skin tethering/nipple retraction not included).

N – Regional lymph nodes
- N0 – No palpable homolateral nodes.
- N1 – Mobile homolateral axillary lymph nodes.
- N2 – Fixed homolateral axillary lymph nodes.
- N3 – Homolateral supra/infraclavicular lymph nodes or oedema of arm.

M – Distant metastasis
- M0 – No distant metastasis.
- M1 – Distant metastasis.

INVESTIGATIONS

i. **Routine**
- Detailed haemogram
  - TLC/DLC
  - Hb%

- ESR
- RBC and platelets count.

- Complete blood chemistry
  - Blood urea
  - Serum creatinine
  - Blood sugar
  - LFT.
- Urine analysis
  - Routine examination (Sugar, albumin ketone bodies)
  - Microscopic examination of urine.
- X-ray chest PA view.
- Ultrasound test of breast (differential diagnosis between cystic and solid lesions).
- FNAC.

ii. **Specialised/optional investigation**

- Mammography of the other breast-to rule out another primary mass or a secondary.
- Isotope scanning of bones: may show bone secondaries much before X-ray film can, particularly valuable in presence of bone pains and negative X-ray films.
- CAT scans.

Management

A. For early stages Stage I and II

- **1st step** is radical mastectomy or extended simple mastectomy. Then depending upon the status of the nodes and histopathology further radiotherapy and chemotherapy (CT) is given.
- If patient is young and disease is very early (Stage I) then only a LUMPECTOMY can be done to be followed by radiotherapy.

B. For Stage III and IV (Advanced Stage)

- Radical surgery cannot be done here. Role of surgery is limited in the form of toilet mastectomy.
- Radiotherapy is the treatment of choice here, radiotherapy is to be followed by CT and/or hormone therapy (HT).

> **Note:** *Treatment of CA breast depend upon the stage and its natural history. Usually treatment is done by surgery/RT/CT/HT depending upon various factors like stage, age of the patient, menopausal status, etc.*

Role of Surgery in Breast C_A

> **Note:** *It is the treatment of choice in early stage of the disease.*

Various types of surgical procedures are undertaken like–

a. **Lumpectomy:** Local excision of tumour. This is done only in very early stage and has to be followed by radiotherapy. Its advantage is that breast can be conserved.

b. **Extended simple mastectomy:** Removal of the complete breast plus nodes in lower axilla. Pectoral muscles are preserved here. It is most commonly done these days.

c. **Radical mastectomy** (Halsted): Whole breast is removed along with pectoral muscles and nodes are cleared as much as possible. One of the disadvantage of this surgery that cosmetically it is poor with postoperative oedema of arm, very common.

d. **Modified radical mastectomy (Patey's)**: Here only pectoralis minor is removed and pectoralis major is left behind along with removal of breast and axillary nodes.

e. **Toilet mastectomy**: Palliative surgery help in removing bulk of disease which is a potential source of metastasis.

Role of Radiotherapy (RT) in C_A Breast

> **Note:** *CA breast is considered to be moderately sensitive to radiotherapy.*

- Traditional radiotherapy plays an important role in C_A breast, supplementary to surgery and usually given after surgery. The purpose of postoperative radiotherapy is to destroy any residual cancer cell in chest wall or in regional nodes so as to keep these areas of potential spread free from growth. Therefore, it is sometime called PROPHYLACTIC radiotherapy.

> ***Note:*** *In the following situations radiotherapy can be delivered as ADJUVANT treatment:*
> *i. Postoperative radical radiotherapy as adjuvant.*
> *ii. Palliative-when disease is very advanced or for painful deposits in bone or for metastasis in brain, etc.*
> *iii. For artificial menopause.*

Radiation Technique for Postoperative Radical Radiotherapy

Since the disease has potential to involve skin in chest wall and spread to regional nodes in axilla, supraclavicular nodes and internal mammary nodes, therefore, the purpose of postoperative radiotherapy is to stabilize any cancer cells residual in chest wall and nodes.

Because of the awakward shapes and curves of area geometrically and the necessity to minimize radiations to lungs, multiple field technique is employed.

Megavoltage or **cobalt beam** is now widely used for its better depth dose and other physical advantages. **Simulator films** should be obtained before executing the treatment planning.

The fields choosen are:

1. Anterior parasternal field: This is done to irradiate the internal mammary nodes. The dose given is usually 5000 r/25 fractions over about 5 weeks usually at about 3 cm depth with 5-6 cm × 15-16 cm covering mammary nodes of both sides.

2. & 3. Fields anterior supraclavicular and axillary field and posterior supraclavicular and axillary field. The dose is calculated at midpoint. The dose delivered is 5000 r/25 fractions over about 5 weeks.

Parasternal and supraclavicular field may be treated separately or in order to avoid junctions by single inverted L-shaped field.

4. & 5. Field lateral tangential field and medial tangential field (or glancing field) in order to irradiate chest wall simultaneously reducing dose to lungs to minimum.

For chest wall, electron is an excellent alternative since electrons have the finite range therefore requisite energy can be used so that the dose to lungs underlying chest wall do not get any radiations.

Important Points

i. Position of the arm of the treatment side: arm is out at about right angle and head in turned to the opposite side.
ii. Take particular care against overdosage or underdosage at field junctions.
iii. Head of humerus and shoulder joint should be shielded properly.
iv. Use adequate bolus.

Reactions may be early or late.

- **Early reaction** is same as discussed above.
- **Late reaction**: with the advent of newer better machines and technologies the reactions are very mild but possibilities are:
  i. Skin scarring and thickening of skin and subcutaneous soft tissue.
  ii. Scarring round the shoulder joint leading to limitation of movement.
  iii. Bone-late necrosis and fracture of ribs, clavicle and upper end of humerus. Not seen now-a-days.
  iv. Lungs: Transient post-radiation pneumonitis especially at apex.

Radiotherapy Following Lumpectomy

- In very early breast C_A following the removal of tumour area (lumpectomy) radical radiotherapy is given to whole breast and drainage area and this is followed by local boost by either using Iridium 192 implant or electron boost (dose 3000 to 5000 rads).

Technique of Artificial Menopause or Ovarian Irradiation

This depends upon age. In younger patient, doses required is more while in older patient dose required is less. Fielding size is usually 15×10 cm^2 with anterior and posterior pelvic fields and doses are calculated at midpoint.

If the patient is nearing menopause, single fraction of 450 rads can induce menopause while in younger patients dose is 1200-1400 rad in 5 to 6 fractions.

CARCINOMA LUNG

Introduction

Lung tumours usually arise in the major bronchus and mediastinal structures.

Lymphatic spread occurs to the lymph nodes of the hilar region of same side and bilaterally to the paratracheal and sub-carinal nodes in mediastinum. Blood-borne metastasis ensues very commonly.

Histological types

Primary	*Secondary*
i. Squamous cell C_A.	i. Breast C_A.
ii. Undifferentiated large cell.	ii. Kidney C_A.
iii. Undifferentiated small cell.	iii. Thyroid C_A.
iv. Adenocarcinoma.	iv. Testis C_A.
v. Alveolar-bronchiolar type.	v. Adrenal C_A.
	vi. Choriocarcinoma.
	vii. Sarcomas.
	viii. Melanoma.

a. Squamous cell C_A

i. Most common variety of lung tumours.
ii. Strong association between squamous cell C_A and smoking.
iii. Usually fast growing.

> ***Note:*** *When present in early stage surgery is the treatment of choice but if the general condition of the patient is not favourable for surgery or the disease is in advanced stages, radiotherapy is the treatment of choice.*

b. Oat cell (small) C_A

i. They are very fast growing tumours.

> ***Note:*** *Even when the primary tumour size is very small, they are considered to have developed micrometastasis, so surgery is usually not done.*

ii. Oat cell C_A is found to be most radiosensitive and chemosensitive.

c. Adenocarcinoma

i. Usually slow growing and seen in the lung periphery.

Evaluation of Patient Having Lung C_A

i. The disease must be defined with the aid of X-ray chest, bronchoscopy, sputum examination for malignant cells, CT scan, etc.

> ***Note:*** *X-ray chest is considered to be the most valuable diagnostic tool for C_A lung and may show abnormal shadow of growth raised diaphragm or erosion of ribs. Along with patient should have complete haematological profile and urine analysis.*

ii. Clinical examination may reveal collapse, consolidation, effusion recurrent laryngeal nerve palsy or extrathoracic spread.

iii. Proper histopathological diagnosis must be sought.

iv. The general condition of the patient should be satisfactory to withstand the radiotherapy.

> ***Note:*** *A large pleural effusion or T.B. in active phase are clear cut contraindications for radiotherapy.*

Treatment: Revolves round 3 things like–

i. Histopathological types of tumour.

ii. Whether the growth is operable or not.
iii. Whether the treatment given is radical or palliative.

ROLE OF SURGERY

As discussed above, surgery is the treatment of choice in few selected cases of squamous cell C_A. It is not done in oat or small cell C_A. Surgery involves lobectomy or pneumonectomy.

> ***Note:*** *Surgery is CONTRAINDICATED in patient of very old age, poor general condition, invasion of mediastinum or chestwall.*

ROLE OF RADIOTHERAPY

- As postoperative.
- As primary mode of treatment modality where surgery is contraindicated or refused.

Principles of Treatment Planning in Lung C_A

A. When planning radical treatment

Careful planning and accurate beam direction are essential as dose to vital nearby structures at risk like normal lung tissue and spinal cord must be kept within tolerance levels. This is accomplished usually by treatment in two phases. The initial phase covers the whole mediastinum including sub carinal nodes. In 2nd phase after 4000 r 20 for the volume is reduced to cover the primary site and same side nodes to a dose of 6000 to 6500 r/30 fraction for radical treatment, a 3 field plan is necessary in order to spare vital structures.

B. For planning of palliative treatment

The volume usually included is primary tumour with margin of about 2 cm mediastinal nodes can be included. The technique is usually simple anterior and posterior parallel and opposed fields are sufficient.

Dose delivered is 3000-3500 rads in 10 fractions or upto 4000 rads depending upon the field size.

FIELD ARRANGEMENT

For three field techniques.

1st phase: Initially parallel opposed fields using anterior and posterior fields are employed.

2nd phase: This is followed by 3 field planning, the lesion can be peripheral or central.

a. If the lesion is **peripheral**, then one anterior field with wedge, one posterior field with wedge and one lateral field is used.
b. For central lesion when treatment volume lies **centrally** in front of spinal cord, an open anterior and two posterior oblique fields with wedge are used to spare spinal cord.

> ***Note:*** *Lung corrections are made for proper dose delivery because air in normal lung impairs tissue penetration. If the beam passes through lung tissue which is aerated, for two posterior oblique fields in Megavoltage, 15% should be added to conventional figures.*

CARCINOMA UTERINE BODY

Introduction

It is a disease of perimenopausal or postmenopausal lady. Most of the patient present are in early stage. Irregular bleeding especially after menopause is the cardinal symptoms.

> ***Note:*** *There is a strong relationship between diabetes mellitus, hypertension, obesity and C_A body of uterus.*

Investigations done

- Complete haemogram
  - TLC/DLC, ESR, Hb%, RBC count.
  - Thrombocytes count, etc.
- Urine analysis.
- Blood sugar.
- Kidney function tests—Blood urea and serum creatinine.
- Liver function tests—Serum bilirubin, SGOT, SGPT, serum alkaline phosphatase.

- VDRL.
- X-ray chest (PA view).
- Cystoscopy.
- Barium enema (optional).
- Lymphangiogram (optional).
- CAT scan (optional), and
- D & C (Dilatation and curettage).

SPREAD OF DISEASE

Treatment

C_A body uterus can invade deep uterine wall and may penetrate parametrium. It may spread downwards. In this situation, it is not possible to comment whether the growth is arising primarily from C_X or body of uterus. Such cases are regarded as C_A C_X. Secondary deposits are commonly seen in ovaries as well as in lower vagina.

Lymph node metastasis to pelvic lymph node also ensues but is less frequent as compared to C_A C_X. From pelvic nodes the disease may spread to para-aortic lymph nodes.

Distant metastasis may occur by bloodstream to lungs, liver, bone, etc.

Various treatment modalities are available and optimum treatment depends upon various factors like stage, general condition of patient, surgical and histological detail like myometrial invasion, whether more than or less than one-third of thickness, grading, etc.

Stage I: Disease confined to uterus.

i. If patient operable: The primary standard treatment is surgery, i.e. total or radical hysterectomy (removal of uterus, ovaries, uterine tubes).

> ***Note:*** *Following surgery, if the disease is associated with favourable prognostic variable like grade I tumour, myometrial invasion less than one-third of thickness and ovaries and tubes not involved then keep the patient for follow-up and no need for any radiotherapy in these cases.*

ii. If following surgery the disease is associated with associated features like grade II/III tumour, poorly differentiated, myometrial invasion more than one-third of thickness then there are chances that these patients are likely to develop recurrence, then patient requires adjuvant treatment by radiotherapy to control micrometastasis.

> ***Note:*** *The radiotherapy is delivered by combination of external radiotherapy and brachytherapy (BT).*

External radiotherapy: 2000 rads in 10 fractions to whole pelvis plus 3000 rads to parametrium. This is followed by intracavitary radiotherapy (vault radium) to prevent vault recurrence.

> ***Note:*** *The total dose to point 'A' should not exceed 8000 rads.*

This is also applied to **Stage II** C_A body of uterus.

iii. If the patient is not fit for surgery owing to some advanced disease then radiotherapy is given as sole modality with a curative intent. Combination of external radiotherapy 2000 rads to whole pelvis plus 3000 rads to parametrium (parametrium with midline block) to be followed by intracavitary brachytherapy in 2 sessions point 'A' should not get more than 8000 rads (usually 7500-8000 mg in insertions).

> ***Note:*** *The same applies to stage II inoperable cases. Stage II is labelled as the disease involving corpus and cervix (C_X).*

Stage III: Extension of disease beyond the C_X but still confined to Pelvis.

As such most of these patients are inoperable and are treated by radiotherapy. Whole pelvis radiotherapy 4000 rads to be followed by Parametri. radiotherapy to 6000 rads. This is to be followed by intracavitary insertion (8000 mg hr) done by two intracavitary insert to ensure high central pelvic dose. Dose to point 'A' should not exceed 8000 rads.

> ***Note:*** *Alternatively, patient can be treated by external radiotherapy alone by four field box technique.*

Stage IV: Extrapelvic metastasis, bladder or rectal involvement. Patient usually inoperable. Palliative radiotherapy given to stop bleeding, discharge, relief of pain.

CARCINOMA CERVIX (C_A C_X)

> ***Note:*** *C_A C_X is the most common malignancy seen in females in India and it constitutes about 25 to 30% of all female cancers.*

Recognised Sign and Symptom of C_A C_X– Abnormal or postmenopausal bleeding, discharge P/V, constipation or urinary disturbances are the complaints.

Investigations–As discussed in C_A body of uterus.

Treatment includes: Currently radiotherapy is regarded to be the mainstay of treatment.

> ***Note:*** *Surgery is only useful in early stages/cases. However in these cases also both radiotherapy and surgery give equal results. The treatment is done as per the stage of the C_A C_X.*

Staging of C_A C_X

Stage 0 : Preinvasive C_A.

Stage I : C_A confined strictly to C_X.

Stage II : Spread of disease beyond C_X either to upper vagina or parametrium but has not reached to lateral pelvic wall.

Stage III : Disease has involved lateral pelvic wall or lower one-third of vagina.

Stage IV : Advanced local growth involving mucosae of urinary bladder or rectum or distant metastasis.

RADIOTHERAPY TECHNIQUES

C_A C_X is treated by both intracavitary brachytherapy (BT) or external radiotherapy, either alone or in combination depending upon various factors like anatomy of pelvis, bulk of disease and the stage.

Teletherapy (TT)

Now-a-days TT or external radiotherapy is given by MEGAVOLTAGE radiation using cobalt-60 machine or linear accelerator.

> ***Note:*** *Orthovoltage or Kilovoltage radiations are not used because of its physical disadvantages.*

Brachytherapy (BT)

> ***Note:*** *In the 1920's and 1930's the treatment of C_A C_X was based on intracavitary Radium.*

There are two techniques of treatment were **Stockholm** and **Paris** technique.

- In **Stockholm technique** higher intensity radium applications of relatively short duration repeated every 2 to 3 weeks.

> ***Note:*** *In fact, it is a high dose fractionated method.*

- In **Paris technique** low intensity radium treatment of upto 1 week duration was used. It is a low dose continuous method.

> ***Note:*** *Both Stockholm and Paris techniques were emperical and not scientific.*

- This was followed by **Manchester method** which defined point 'A' and calculations were based on predetermined point 'A' and point 'B'.
- **Point 'A'**– is regarded as critical point. It is a point 2 cm above and 2 cm lateral to the lower most radioactive source in cervix (C_X).

> ***Note:*** *At this point artery crosses the ureter and maximum tolerance is 5000 rads.*

- **Point 'B'**– It is situated 3 cm lateral to point 'A'.
- BT can be executed by pre-loaded applications or it can be done by after loading techniques. After loading can be either manual or remote control after loading.

Treatment According to Stage of the Disease (C_A C_X)

1. In Stage I and early Stage II

a. If the disease is small then 1st brachytherapy (intracavitary insertion) is given in two sessions, each session of 4000 rads in 72 hours with a gap of one week.

> ***Note:*** *By this method point 'A' gets 8000 rads.*

- Since in India follow up of patient is not satisfactory so it is advised to give 3500 rads/ 15 fractions by central shielding using anterior and posterior fields.

b. If the disease is bulky at initial presentation, then policy is to deliver external radiotherapy first (4000/4 weeks) an after a gap of 3 to 4 weeks. One single session of intracavitary insertion is given (4000 r in 72 hours).

2. In Advanced stage

> ***Note:*** *Radiotherapy is the treatment of 1st choice (TO1C).*

- Here initially external radiotherapy is given to whole pelvis (4500) rads/4 and 4½ weeks in 20 fractions) followed by anterior and posterior parallel and opposed fields. After a gap of about 4 weeks. Single session of intercavitary radiotherapy is given with dose to point A being 3500 rads, therefore overall dose to point 'A' by external and intracavitary therapy remains within tolerance limits.

3. **Stage IV**- external radiotherapy by four field "**box**" technique 4000 to 4500 rads/20-22 fractions.
4. In patients which are suitable for BT it is advisable to give only external radiotherapy by four field technique by employing anterior pelvic field, posterior pelvic field, left lateral pelvic field and right lateral pelvic field.

Geometry of field

Centre is roughly taken at a point 3 cm above border of pubic symphisis. Around this a field of 15 × 15 cm^2 is drawn. In lateral fields, the centre should be at greater trochanter, and around this a field of 8 × 15 cm^2 is drawn. Simulator film is always taken before executing the treatment.

Technique of Intracavitary Insertion

Previously **radium** used to be employed but presently it has been discarded in favour of **caesium**.

> ***Note:*** *The aim of intracavitary therapy is to deliver very high dose to central tumour bearing area without exceeding the tolerance of surrounding sensitive organs like rectum and urinary bladder.*

Tolerance of various organs includes:

Rectum	6500 rads
Urinary bladder	7000 rads
Point 'A'	8000 rads.

- Radiation insertion is carried out in operation theatre (OT) under general anaesthesia (GA). The C_X is gently and gradually dilated using a series of metal dilators of increasing length.

  The length of ureters measured using a **uterine sound** and the width of the vaginal vault is assessed.

> ***Note:*** *The average uterine canal (C_X and body) is about 6 cm long.*

- Manchester technique or BAARC technique is usually used for caesium insertion using a uterine tendem and vaginal voids. Sources are inserted with the help of long forceps.

Loading of Sources

It is the distribution or assembly of source in such a way that dose to point 'A' remains same. Any combination of activities can be used. The aim is to insert the longest tube and longest ovoids that the cavities allow.

Standardized application is:

i. Ovoids–made in 3 sizes for small or large vaults 9 units (long), 8 units (medium), 7 units (small).

ii. Tube: Long–6 units, 4 units 4 units (two). Medium –6 units, 4 units (Two), Small–5 units.

> ***Note:*** *1 unit = 2.5 mg of radium.*

- When the applicators have been inserted, the vagina is packed with gauze. By packing the dose to rectum and bladder gets reduced.

  Dose rate is 56.7 rads/hour to 57.6 rads/hour. Following insertion of applicators the patient is taken to X-ray department. Where AP and lateral film are taken and inspected by RADIO–THERAPIST and only if the distribution is satisfactory the actual radioactive sources are inserted.

> ***Note:*** *Patients are nursed in radiation protected room while sources are in position. After the pre-calculated time is over, sources are removed.*

- **Scintillation counter** may be inserted in rectum at the end of the procedure and the maximum dose rate at the rectal mucosae is obtained by a series of readings at various distance along the rectal wall. If the dose is found excessive the radioactive sources must be readjusted. It is also possible to insert the probe via urethra into the bladder and measure the dose at the bladder base.

Patient Care

Patient may develop symptoms like diarrhoea, increased urinary frequency, skin reactions manifesting as acute radiation reaction. Patient is reassured and given symptomatic treatment with adequate fluid intake.

> ***Note:*** *For skin reactions Gention Violet (G.V.) paint is used.*

SEMINOMA TESTIS (ST)

Important Considerations at a Glance

- The tumour ST spreads in orderly fashion. It has a considerable importance in the treatment policy.
- The lymphatics of testis follow the spermatic vessels and end in the group of nodes round the abdominal aorta at the level of renal veins (Para-aortic nodes).

> **Note:** *Common iliac nodes may also be involved.*

- From abdomen the lymphatic channels extend up through the mediastinum and finally supraclavicular nodes may be involved.

> **Note:** *Inguinal nodes are only involved when scrotal sac is invaded by tumour or when FNAC procedure is done to know the tumour type.*

- **Spread** by blood usually ensues to lung which is rather more common in **Non-seminomatous tumours**.

Classification

a. Seminomatous tumorus–They are most common testicular tumours and affects males of 30 to 50 years age groups.

> **Note:** *These tumours are highly radiosensitive.*

b. **Non-seminomatous tumours** affect males of 15 to 40 years age group. They can be of following types like–
   - Teratoma.
   - Embryonal cell C_A.
   - Choriocarcinoma.

> **Note:** *Non-seminomatous tumours are not very radiosensitive, so the dose required to treat these tumours is more.*

Sign and Symptom Includes

- First symptom is gradually enlarging painless testicular swelling but 1st symptom may be cause of secondary deposits in lungs leading to respiratory symptoms or para-aortic lymphadenopathy presenting as lump abdomen or obstructive symptoms.

Evaluation of the Patient

- In addition to usual extent of disease evaluation and assessment of general medical and nutritional status, these patient should have IVP, lymphangiogram, tumour markers, α-fetoproteins and hCG levels.

Investigation Includes

- Complete blood counts (CBC).
- Chest X-ray.
- Blood chemistry–urea, sugar, serum electrolytes, etc.
- R/E of urine/microscopic.
- IVP.
- Lymphangiography.
- Tumour markers—α-Fetoprotein, hCG levels.

Treatment Includes

1. Surgery–First orchidectomy. It removes tumour and provides its histopathological diagnosis.
2. Radiotherapy (RT)–Since tumour is highly radiosensitive. Treatment depends upon the stage.

Stage I • Disease confined to testis and spermatic cord.

Radiotherapy Treatment

- Elective radiation of para-aortic and ipsilateral pelvic region by anterior and posterior parallel opposing L-shaped fields. Great care is taken to almost exclude both the kidneys.
- In the anterior field, the pelvic portion is larger to include the orchidectomy scar and adjoining inguinal lymphatics.
- The portal extends upwards to include the pelvic nodes to lower border of L_4 (as checked by simulator) thereafter

including the para-aortic nodes and ipsilateral renal hilum upto centre of T_{11}.

- The lower border of anterior field is at lower border of symphysis pubis and of the posterior field at sacrococcygeal junction.

Stage II : Disease is beyond testis but is confined below diaphragm.

Stage III: Supradiaphragmatic extension. Treatment is done in two phases.

Phase I 3/4 whole abdomen plus pelvis radiotherapy-field size is that, upper limit is dome of diaphragm while lower border is inferior border of obturator foramen. Dose- 3000 rads/4-5 weeks. (150 rads daily).

Phase II treatment

In stage II (elective) and stage II (therapeutic) of whole mediastinum and both supraclavicular regions through parallel opposing 'T' shaped fields, after 2 weeks from completion of abdomen-pelvic (phase I) course, dose is 2600 rads/13 fractions.

Precautions to be taken

a. The other testis is schielded properly and dose is monitored by TLD dosimetry.
b. Treatment should be suspended temporarily if there is a marked bone marrow depression (TLC count below 2000 or platelets below 80000/cmm) or if there is a severe diarrhoea.

Other Testicular Tumours

The radiotherapy dose is higher around 4000/25 fraction-27 fraction.

There is a greater role of surgery and chemotherapy.

> ***Note:*** *A considerable amount of bone marrow, pelvis and vertebrae lies within the treated volume and blood counts should be done twice weekly.*

CARCINOMA LOWER PHARYNX, LARYNX AND POSTCRICOID

- Lower pharynx extends from tip of epiglottis to the lower end of cricoid cartilage at the junction of hypopharynx and oesophagus.
- Larynx is grouped under these parts.
    - i. **Glottis** area bearing vocal cords.
    - ii. **Supraglottic** area lies above glottis.
    - iii. **Infraglottic** area lies below glottis.

Pathology: Majority of them are squamous cell C_A.

Sign and Symptom (S/S): Depending upon the site and extent of the disease the patient may have **hoarseness of voice, dyspnoea, dysphagia** or lump in the neck (cervical adenopathy).

> ***Note:*** *In the advanced stage the patient may have stridor, i.e. audible wheezing on inspiration and is an impending emergency.*

Investigations

Patient should be evaluated thoroughly by local clinical examination, indirect and direct laryngoscopy, where indicated X-ray soft tissue neck for local extent of disease, X-ray chest for any spread of disease on lungs. In addition patient should also undergo complete haematological profile.

Treatment is divided into 2 headings:

a. **General:** Improving the general condition of the patient by giving high protein diet, haematinic, and vitamins.

> ***Note:*** *Ryles tube is put in patient who have dysphagia and tracheostomy is done in advance cases when indicated.*

b. **Specific:** In early cancer case, patient can be managed by either surgery or radiotherapy, both giving similar result. But in surgery there is loss of voice, apart from this radical operations are drastic and mutilating and patient has permanent tracheostomy. The emphasis is put on radiation use.

Radiation technique applied depends upon the stage and extent of disease. As such dosage to the spinal cord must be kept within limits of tolerance.

In early growth of larynx confined strictly to glottis localized radiotherapy by a small field of 6 × 6 cm or 7 × 7 cm by using anterior pair is employed. This technique gives wedge excellant high dose distribution to larynx. The dose given 6000 rads/30 for over 6 weeks by megavoltage.

For supraglottic and pharyngeal growth since they are liable to be locally invasive and develop metastasis to regional nodes early therefore the nodes are also included in the treatment of field and large fields are used therefore lateral parallel opposed fields are employed including nodal areas, care must be taken that posterior edge of the field is clear of spinal cord.

Dose given is 6000 rads in 6 to 7 weeks.

Postcricoid cancer usually presents with dysphagia. These tumours are managed as cancer of upper third of oesophagus.

CARCINOMA OF HEAD AND NECK

Carcinoma Oral Cavity

Introduction

It is the most common cancer seen in India.

Aetiology

Commonly responsible aetiological factors include–

- Poor dental hygiene.
- Sharp tooth.
- Tobacoo.
- Syphilis, etc.
- Alcohol.

Leukoplakia is defined as the white patch on oral mucosa measuring 5 cm or more which cannot be scrapped off and which cannot be attributed to any other diagnostic condition sites– Buccal mucosa, upper and lower alveolus, and gingival tongue, floor mouth, hard palate.

Histologically most of the C_A oral cavity is squamous cell C_A, others include–Lymphoepithelioma and C_A tonsil.

Clinical Presentation

They usually present as ulcer, fissure or nodule leukoplakia may be present. The lesion may extend locally to involve other sites of oral cavity.

> **Note:** *In advanced stage there may be tongue fixity, bone involvement, skin involvement and patient may have otalgia (ear ache), slurred speech, excessive salivation or trismus.*

Spread of disease

There may be local, nodal and haematogenous spread. The predominant nodes involved are submandibular nodes, upper deep cervical nodes, mid cervical and lower deep cervical nodes in advanced stage.

Staging – done by TNM staging system.

T : Primary tumour

T_{1S} : Carcinoma *in situ*.

T_1 : Tumour 1 cm or less.

T_2 : Tumour > 2 cm but < 4 cm.

T_3-T_4 : Locally very advanced disease involving nearby structures with fixity of tongue, involvement of bone or skin.

N_0 : No palpable nodes.

N_1 : Involvement of nodes of same side but nodes are mobile.

N_2 : Mobile bilateral nodes or contralateral nodes.

N_3 : Fixed nodes.

M_0 : No evidence of distant metastasis.

M_1 : Distant metastasis seen.

Treatment

> **Note:** *The chief curative modes of treatment remain surgery and radiotherapy.*

- In early and moderately advanced lesions similar results are obtained with each method.

- Radiotherapy is usually preferred because of the preservation of function and minimum morbidity.

> ***Note:*** *Surgery is preferred in selected situation like CA tip of the tongue, syphilitic base, etc.*

Radiotherapy (RT)

The radiation technique depends on the site and size of the growth as well as the presence of nodal secondaries.

i. **Early stage**

In early stage (upto 4 cm), interstitial irradiation affords the best method. The anterior two-third of tongue is one of the few sites in the body where interstitial methods still retain their place as the treatment of choice.

- Interstitial implant may in the form of single implant eradicating effectively a slab of tissue 1 cm thick or two implant or multiple implant depending upon the size and thickness of the lesion.
- The implant may be **temporary** (e.g. Radium or its substitute like ^{60}Cobalt, Caesium^{137}, and Iridium^{192}) or **permanent** (in thin isotope having short half-life are used and the source is allowed to decay to inactivity in the tissue implanted as gold^{198} such with a half-life of 2.7 days).

Dose: A typical dose is 6000 rads in 6 days. Similarly early lesion can be treated by interstitial brachytherapy in floor of mouth, buccal mucosa, etc.

ii. **Advanced lesions radical treatment**

For lesions unsuitable for implantation, mega-voltage or cobalt beam is used and the technique and field size depends upon the size and position of the growth as well as on the status of regional cervical nodes, whether they are palpable or fixed.

Usually a simple parallel pair is satisfactory for most cases to give a tumour dose of about 6500 rads in about 6.5 to 7 weeks.

While planning it should be kept in mind that whole of the primary is included in the radiation field. If upper deep cervical nodes are involved then the field includes the nodes of next station because of the chances of micrometastasis.

> ***Note:*** *While delivering radiation it should be noted that spinal cord should not get the dose beyond its tolerance (4500 rads).*

- In case of C_A base of tongue or tonsil, whole of the neck is treated because high chances of lymph node involvement.
- For anterior two-third of tongue, floor of mouth, hard palate the superior margin of the field is usually at the level of mastoid tip and for C_A of posterior one-third tongue, tonsil, soft palate, the superior margin is usually at the zygomatic because these organs, according to surface anatomy lies at the level of angle of mandible.

  The patient should be treated in supine position with neck extended which will help in pushing the nodes more anteriorly in case of C_A tonsil and buccal mucosa.

  When the disease is in early stage and localized to one tonsil without crossing the midline, the dose can be delivered by 2:1 loading for floor of mouth, alveolus wedge may be used depending upon the position of lesion.

Booster dose is given by giving high dose in smaller field accompanying initial area of gross disease. In order to spare spinal cord, boost can be given by electron beam because of its property of having a finite range.

For regional nodes 5000 rads/5 weeks is sufficient to eradicate micrometastasis in clinically negative nodes.

Lymphatic (Nodes) Metastasis in Neck

> ***Note:*** *Presence or absence of cervical nodes has a strong hold on the possible outcome of the disease.*

- In general, it is usually considered that mobile nodes which are operable nodes in squamous C_A are best treated by surgery in the form of radical neck dissection, while fixed nodes which are considered inoperable may be treated by external radiotherapy and are included in the radiation field along with primary lesion as discussed above.

  In head and neck, there are 3 clinical situations.

1. **No nodes palpable:**
   Here according to some oncologist prophylactic neck dissection of nodes undertaken owing to possible risk of micrometastasis or early secondaries, etc.

   > ***Note:*** *Majority of oncologists prefer "wait and watch" policy by which patients undergoing regular and meticulous follow-up when nodes are apparant they may be considered for surgery.*

2. **Palpable nodes:**
   i. Some prefer irradiate the primary 1st and when reactions subside, consider the patient for surgery.
   ii. Others prefer to remove the ndoes 1st and then advocate radiotherapy.
   iii. Rest who prefer to treat primary surgically and remove both primary and lymph nodes in one session.

   > ***Note:*** *In cases where surgery is contraindicated for radical neck dissection, radiotherapy is used.*

3. **Fixed Nodes:**
   Here due to affection of lymph node capsule it become fixed so Radical Neck dissection is not feasible in such cases. So here they are treated along with primary by radiotherapy alone.

Radiation Reactions

Patients are advised to forbid SMOKING, ALCOHOL intake and TOBACCO chewing (Khaini) and spicy food. By the end of 2nd week of the course of radiotherapy, mucosal reactions usually begin to appear, they are redness of skin, ulceration, etc.

- It is always a strain on any patient with soreness, loss of taste and dysphagia. At this time proper hygiene and nutritions should be ensured frequent mouth wash. Local anaesthetic suspension may be taken.
- After the phase of acute reaction is over, late effects follow. There is dryness of mouth and owing to radiation to parotids which are included in the radiation field, loss of taste sensation is another effect, but usually recovers.
- Skin changes including EPILATION are generally mild with megavoltage.
- There can be late dental complications but less pronounced than in era of kilovoltage radiations when bony necrosis of mandible used to be the much pronounced.

TUMOURS OF THE CNS (BRAIN)

Introduction

CNS tumours are either primary or secondary.

> ***Note:** Most common tumour metastasizing to CNS comes from BREAST, LUNG, KIDNEY, etc.*

- They may occur in children as well as adult so no age is exempted.
- They are classified according to their tissue of origin.

Signs and Symptoms

Usually CNS tumours present with headache (waking up in the morning), vomiting and papilloedema. There can be weakness in limbs, epileptic fits, visual field defects and as the disease progresses there may be drowsiness, and mental retardation. The localizing signs depends upon the primary site of tumour.

As for example:

- Cerebellar lesion : Incoordination and ataxia.
- Brainstem lesion : Cranial Nerve palsy.
- Temporal lobe lesion : Disorder of language.
- Pituitary lesion : Gigantism or acrome–galy.

Table 14.1: Classification of CNS Tumours

Cell types	*Histological types*	*Comments if any*
1. Meninges	Meningioma	Usually benign.
2. Neuroglial	• Glioma	Common glioma tumour.
	• Astrocytoma	Graded into four grades from benign to highly malignant (Glioblastoma multiformae).
	• Oligodendroglioma	Usually seen in adult.
	• Ependymoma • Medulloblastoma	Childhood tumour, cerebellar in origin, highly malignant and seed via CSF, radiosensitive.
3. Pituitary gland	• Chromophobe adenoma • Eosinophilic adenoma • Basophilic adenoma.	
4. Pineal gland	Pinealoma.	
5. Developmental	Craniopharyngiomas.	
6. Spinal cord tumours	• Intradural intra-medullary	• Ependymoma. • Astrocytoma.
	• Intradural extramedullary	• Schwannomas. • Usually meta-static.
	• Extramedullary.	

Recognised Investigations

- Patient should be thoroughly investigated by taking.
- X-ray skull exhibitng– Feature of:
  - Raised ICP (intracranial pressure)

  - Enlargement of sella turcica or
  - Calcification.
- EEG
- LP and examination of CSF (Raised protein, etc).
- CAT/MRI scan.
- Angiography.
- Pneumoencephalography.

Treatment

Surgery the treatment of choice, but practically it may not be possible and many times only biopsy is possible and where biopsy also is not feasible owing to complex structure of brain radiotherapy in the form of primary treatment or postoperative treatment is usually advocated.

Radiation technique depends upon the type of tumour, the site and the radiation tolerance. Before starting the radiation treatment the raised ICP should always be relieved by basic steroids, etc. because radiation is likely to exacerbate this.

For whole brain treatment simple parallel and opposed fields are used, the dosage are usually 3500 rads in 10 fractions or the equivalent in longer lines. Smaller fields, e.g. to the brainstem, can be given 5000 rads in 5 weeks.

Note: *For spinal cord tumours if the length upto 15 cm is treated then dose should not exceed 3500 rads in 3 weeks though shorter lengths can be given upto 4000 rads.*

Whole CNS Axis Radiation

This is indicated in condition where whole neurospinal axis is at risk of medulloblastoma, ependymoma, pinealoma. These tumours have the tendency to seed in CSF, therefore, special technique is being required to cover the whole cerebrospinal axis.

Several techniques are available employing MEGAVOLTAGE rads following surgery (removing a part of growth), separate fields for skull and spine are used.

- For skull, two lateral parallel and opposed fields are applied and this includes spine down to 2nd cervical vertebra. Dosage is 4000 rads in 4 weeks; followed by boost to posterior fossa (True site of primary growth) by small field in 500 rads. The overall treatment is planned for about 5 weeks.
- The rest of spine is covered by a field upto 3rd sacral vertebra (where spinal dura ends). To avoid excessive dosage at the junction, a gap of 0.5 cm is left between the margins of the field.
- The spinal field is further divided into two fields of un-equal length alternating the fields everyday. This is done so that effect of inhomogenous dosage at field junction are minimised.

> **Note:** *In case where the child is non co-operative, restless, general anaesthesia is given before each treatment.*

Reaction

With the advent of megavoltage radiations and proper shielding the reactions have been considerably reduced. Constitutional reaction may be seen in mild form. Blood counts are advised to be done weekly and if TLC drops below 2000/cmm or platelets below 80,000/cmm then treatment should be temporarily stopped. There will be skin reaction. There will be loss of hair but they re-grow in 2 to 3 months time.

> **Note:** *There may be some late effects in vertebral growth with slight but significant shortening of height in children.*

Tumours of Pituitary Gland

> **Note:** *Pituitary gland govern the functions of other glands like gonads, adrenals and thyroid as well as it has a control over functions.*

Technically pituitary tumours are benign but since they produce local pressure symptoms in brain and optic nerve they are considered **locally malignant**. In addition to the pressure symptoms their growth can cause hormonal upsets in the body by either under or over production of hormones.

CLASSIFICATION

- **Chromophobe adenomas** usually cause pressure symptoms leading to feature of hypopituitarism (hormone deficiencies). They do not produce any secretion.
- **Eosinophil adenoma**: Eosinophilic cells produce hormones that control growth. Therefore an adenoma leading to over growth of these cells will lead to excessive secretions of growth hormone.

> ***Note:*** *In a child who is still in the process of active skeletal growth this may lead to "GIGANTISM" resulting in overgrowth of skeleton while in adults where skeletal growth is complete, the resultant disease is called acromegaly leading to thickening of hands and feet, protruding of the jaw, broadening of nose, coarsening of the features, etc.*

- **Basophil adenoma**: Basophilic cells produce hormone that control the sexual functions and other processes. There may be menstrual disturbances in woman.

Treatment

Surgery or radiotherapy or both.

- **Hypophysectomy**, because complete tumour removal is not possible therefore postoperative radiotherapy is given.
- **Radiotherapy techniques**: Three field (one anterior and two lateral) or four oblique MEGA-VOLTAGE fields above orbit are used.

  The dose is 4500-5000 rads/5 weeks.
- **Brachytherapy**: Yittrium implant, by producing very high dosage locally produces excellent results.
- **Intragamial metastases** are very common. They present with feature of raised ICP and there are

localizing signs depending upon the site of metastasis.

- **Radiotherapy (RT)**: Whole brain is considered to be at risk and therefore the treatment is directed towards whole brain. Parallel and opposed fields are used with field size about 15 × 14 cm giving a dose of about 3000 to 5000 rads over 3 weeks.

> **Note:** *Further treatment depends upon the primary site, e.g. in breast along with hormonal treatment can be started and after this patient can be taken up for chemotherapy.*

Tumours of Orbit Including Eye

> **Note:** *The globe, rectus muscles optic nerve and connective tissue lie in a pyramidal space within the bony walls of orbit.*

- True lymphatics are present only in the eyelids, conjunctiva and lacrimal gland draining primarily to the preauricular and submaxillary nodes, wide variety of tumours both benign and malignant arise from these structures.

Assessment of Primary Orbital Tumour

- Both orbits are examined for any palpable tumour and signs of proptosis or displacement of globe.
- The appearance of the fundus, visual acuity, visual fields and eye movements are assessed.
- Cranial nerve function is tested and the nose and nasopharynx examined for tumour extension.
- The neck is palpated to exclude lymphatic movement, particularly of the preauricular and upper deep cervical nodes, plain X-ray are taken to look for any evidence of bony erosion.
- US and CAT scan help in delineating the soft tissue extension of orbital tumours.

Role of Radiotherapy (RT)

> **Note:** *Radiotherapy plays very vital role in treating wide range of eye and orbital tumours.*

- These tumours may be treated either by brachytherapy or external radiotherapy on the basis of type of tumour and extent of disease.

> ***Note:*** *Many benign conditions like pterygium and corneal vascularisation and squamous cell epitheliomas are treated effectively by strontium 90 applicators.*

- **Lymphomas** may involve the conjunctiva, lacrimal gland and orbit as a part of manifestations of disseminated disease and radiotherapy is employed in these cases to reduce distressing proptosis and diplopia.
- Eyelid lesions especially basal cell C_A may be effectively treated with radiations.
- Metal contact cones are used to protect the eye when these lesions are treated with superficial or deep X-ray therapy.

Retinoblastoma is a most common heritable tumour of childhood. It is an autosomal dominantly inherited tumour. It is bilateral in about 25% of cases.

> ***Note:*** *This is a disease of childhood mainly affecting children around the age of two years.*

Pathology

It arises from the primitive retinal cells invading retina and other tissues of the eye. Its chief route of spread is via optic nerve from where it may invade cranial nerve and brain.

> ***Note:*** *Distant metastasis is also common.*

Clinical Feature

The classical sign of the disease is cat's eye appearance created by an opaque light reflex in normally dark pupil.

Treatment

Principle considerations in treatment planning depend upon whether there is vision or any potential for vision, whether the tumour is confined to globe or there is extension to optic nerve or whether there is orbital, CNS or haematogenous extension.

> ***Note:*** *When the disease is limited to globe choice of therapy depends upon size, location and number of lesions.*

- Most children with unilateral tumour have advanced disease when it is detected often with little or no potential to vision. In such cases ENUCLEATION is the treatment of choice.
- Optic nerve should be removed as great length as possible and carefully examined if nerve is found to contain malignant cells. Postoperative radiotherapy is given to the orbit and the region of nerve stump.
- Presently for unilateral cases when the diagnosis is made at an early stage and there is a great potential for preservation of vision, the concept is that before going in for enucleation, alternative treatment is justified in the form of photocoagulation, cryotherapy or radiotherapy in an attempt to save vision. If there is a failure only then one should go in for surgery.
- After enucleation, patient with residual optic nerve involvement should be given orbital and optic nerve irradiation in dose of 5000 to 5500 rads in 5 to 6 weeks. One of the technique is using a cobalt beam wedge pair.

Management of bilateral disease depends upon extent and group of disease in each eye independently. For managing these lesion there are various schools of thought.

> ***Note:*** *One of the policy which is widely accepted is that lesser affected eye is preserved and other eye which is more severely affected is removed surgically. Efforts are directed towards preservation of the vision of the preserved eye.*

- Of lately thinking has been shifted from surgical treatment to the conservative treatment. It is believed that if useful vision is present in both eyes then neither eye should be enucleated and both should be irradiated because the growth is considered to sensitive to radiations.

> ***Note:*** *Various techniques employing brachytherapy or teletherapy are used and the aim is to treat the entire retina and potential area of disease without producing cataract formation.*

External Radiotherapy

- One of the techniques using an anterior field with divergent lens block together with lateral field.
- The other technique is 'D' shaped lateral field (for unilateral treatment) or opposed lateral field (for bilateral treatment). The D-shaped field is contoured to include entire retinal surfaces and vitreous plus 10 mm of anterior optic nerve while protecting lens to prevent cataract formation. The child should be anaesthesized and immobilized in a reproducible fashion.

Brachytherapy

- Tumour is irradiated by using cobalt disc. In this technique, the eyeball is exposed surgically and a disc holding radioactive cobalt is sutured abutting the tumour mass.

> ***Note:*** *The tumour is the immediate vicinity gets very high dose about 20,000 rads.*

- This technique is useful only for small solitary growth and not for multicentric growth which is usually the case with retinoblastoma.
- The other disadvantages are that it does not treat the whole retina and dose is in homogenous and tissue immediate to source getting very high dose may cause vascular injury.

RENAL TUMOURS

Introduction

Renal tumours may occur in both children and adults.

A. **Renal cell C_A or hypernephroma** is the tumour arising from the renal parenchyma and seen commonly in adults.

Clinical feature: Typically presents as haematuria, flank pain and abdominal mass (a classical triad).

Other clinical features may be seen like fever and polycythemia.

Management includes detailed clinical examination and detailed investigations like complete haemogram, detailed serum chemistry which includes kidney and liver function, complete urine analysis, IVP, X-ray chest and imaging techniques like CT scan and renal angiogram.

Treatment: Surgery is the main treatment.

Role of radiotherapy: To be used as pre-operatively or postoperatively or for palliative treatment.

Preoperative radiotherapy: May improve resectability in cases which are inoperable.

Postoperative radiotherapy: Where tumour is very extensive at the time of surgery, or if tumour ruptures.

Field: As choosen by simulator.

Anteriorly-superior border-diaphragm, **inferior border**-iliac crest, **medially**-contralateral paravertebral gutter short of contralateral kidney.

An anteroposterior localization film is taken care must be taken to exclude other kidney by IVP. Anteroposterior parallel opposed portal are used.

Dose: 4500-5000 rads 4½ to 5 weeks.

When tumour is bilateral (both kidneys contain tumour).

The basic approach is removal of the kidney on the more involved side. Radiotherapy is given along with CT at the site of nephrectomy as well as to the remaining kidney. The remaining kidney receives a dose of 1400 rads, after which it is excluded from radiation field. The renal bed of nephrectomy is given a further dose upto 2000 rads.

- WBC and platelets may show improvement.
- Growth of vertebrae may show shortening.

B. **Wilms' tumour or nephroblastoma** is a tumour of childhood. It arises from neoplastic changes in developmental malformation of kidney from ectodermal and mesodermal tissues.

Treatment is usually a combination of surgery, radiotherapy and CT.

Clinical feature: The age varies from few months to 10 years but most children are below 5 years. Classic presentation is large swelling in flank usually noticed by parents. Full treatment assessment should be made by various haematological and radiological investigations which include both conventional and imaging technique like IVP, isotopic whole body scan, CT scan, etc.

Pattern of Spread of Disease

The growth spread rapidly locally leading to invasions and adhesions. Lymphatic spread already ensues to para-aortic nodes.

Distant metastasis by bloodstream usually occurs in lungs, liver and bone. It may presents as bilateral disease in about 10% of cases.

Treatment

Surgery (Nephrectomy) is the 1st step in the management of Wilm's tumour. After the surgery the further treatment depends upon stage and histopathological types whether belonging to favourable or unfavourable histology.

Radiotherapy (RT)

When the tumour is small-radiotherapy is given to tumour bed and regional nodes, by employing parallel and opposed anterior and posterior fields using cobalt (Co-60) beam. The field extends from dome of diaphragm to sacral promontory and medial boundary is extended across the midline to include entire vertebrae. The other kidney is carefully shielded as seen by IVP. The tumour doses are usually about 2000 rads over 2 weeks.

> ***Note:*** *Following surgery it is advisable to start radiotherapy within 48 hours.*

Treatment for Locally Massive Disease

Whole abdomen radiotherapy is given from pelvic floor to diaphragm. Femoral heads are shielded so that not to interfere with the skeletal growth. The opposite kidney is shielded from the beginning. The given dose is 2000 rads over 3 weeks.

> ***Note:*** *When disease is very advanced and has involved lungs or liver, following is the line of treatment.*

Involvement of Lungs

Lungs are included in their entirety in the radiation field which also encompasses the renal bed on the involved side upto dose of 1400 rads. After this radiotherapy is continued to renal bed for additional dose.

Metastasis to Liver

Dose should be given 2000 rads in 2 weeks.

For Bilateral Tumours

The basic approach is removal of the kidney on the more involved side. Radiotherapy is given along with chemotherapy to the site of Nephrectomy as well as to the remaining kidney. The remaining kidney receives a dose of 1400 rads after which it is excluded from radiation field. The renal bed is given further dose upto 2000 rads.

Radiation reactions seen during radiotherapy is GIT irritation (nausea and vomiting). There can be haematological toxicity affected WBC and platelet count. In the long run, patient may have vertebrae growth impairment leading to shortening of effective height of the patient treated.

C_A **urinary bladder** seen in aniline dye workers, smokers (tobacco) and most common histological type is transitional cell C_A.

Management includes all investigation as done for testicular tumours plus includes bimanual examination under general anaesthesia with cystoscopic biopsy done for staging and histopathology.

Role of radiotherapy can be:

a. Preoperative radiotherapy.
b. Radical radiotherapy.
c. Palliative radiotherapy.

a. **Preoperative radiotherapy** given to all patient where surgery (cystectomy) is planned.

   Field: Whole pelvis irradiation including the urinary bladder and pelvic nodes.

   > ***Note**: Anterior and posterior parallel opposing portals are used and average field is 15 × 15 cm to 16 × 16 cm. The field extends from upper border fo L5 to ischial tuberosities and at mid acetabula laterally.*

   Dose: 2000 rads mid depth in 5 to 6 fraction daily using megavoltage radiation.

b. **Radical Radiation Therapy**

   Field should be decided by simulator.

   Simulation: With patient lying supine on simulation table, Foley's catheter is inserted and 20 ml of UROGRAFIN and 20 ml of air is introduced into bladder cavity.

   An antero-posterior film is taken and marked on the skin delineating the whole pelvis from upper border of L_3 to below obturator foramina and at the centre of acetabular lateral to bony pelvic brims, 40 ml of barium is injected into the rectum by a catheter syringe with its tip inside the anus.

> ***Note:*** *Lateral film is taken to delineate urinary bladder and rectum.*

- Radical radiotherapy can be delivered by 360° rotation therapy, 4 field box technique,- anterior field/and two lateral wedge fields.
- **Dose**: Initial whole pelvis radiotherapy to 4000 rads/20 fractions mid depth dose in 4 weeks. Then 2000 to 2500 rads to bladder region in 2 to 2½ weeks using multiple field technique for a total dose of 6000 to 6500 in 6 to 6½ weeks.

c. **Palliative Radiotherapy**

For patients who are unsuitable for radical radiotherapy, or having poor general condition or having **massive uncontrolled haematuria**.

Field: Anterior and posterior parallel opposing pelvic portal about 12 × 12 cm.

Dose: Mid plane dose of 2000 rads in 5 fractions.

> ***Note:*** *All patients should be instructed to empty his urinary bladder prior to each treatment.*

DERMA/SKIN/CUTIS CARCINOMA

Types of Skin C_A

a. **Squamous cell C_A or epidermoid C_A**–It can manifest anywhere in skin.

> ***Note:*** *Factors predisposing to squamous cell C_A (SCC).*

- Senile keratosis.
- Sun, X-rays exposure.
- Bowen's disease.
- Pitch, coal tar, soot, smoking.
- Lupus vulgaris.
- Marjolin's ulcer.

b. **Basal cell C_A or rodent ulcer**– Its commonest site is over face. It presents as an ulcer with raised margins. The tumour is very slowly growing and usually remains localized.

> ***Note:*** *Recognised features of basal cell CA.*

- About 90% seen on the face.
- Rolled pearly edge appearance.
- Central ulceration with scabbing.
- Treatment involves local excision, or irradiation therapy (RT).

c. **Melanoma:** It is a rapidly growing tumour biologically very-very aggressive. It spreads by lymphatics as well as by blood-stream.

Differential diagnosis of malignant malanoma

- From benign naevae: Intradermal-compound-Juvenile-junctional.
- Seborrheic keratosis.
- Sclerosing angioma.
- Pyogenic granuloma.
- Pigmented basal cell C_A.

Q. Which pigmented lesions should be excised?

- Any mole undergoing charge.
- Naevae in areas subjected to trauma.
- Black moles > 0.5 cm in diameter especially leg/back.
- Naevae on soles of feet, mucosa, genitalia, etc.
- Moles on anxious patient with bad family history.
- Children with solitary growing mole.
- Those causing cosmetic problems.

Recognised signs of malignant transformation

- Increase in size.
- Increase in colour (Pigmentation).
- Areas of depigmentation.
- Ulceration or bleeding.
- Irritation.
- Satellite lesions and spread of pigment from edge of lesion.
- Regional lymph node enlargement-distant metastasis.

d. **Mycosis fungoides**–T cell lymphoma.
e. **Secondary carcinoma of skin**– usually seen as a nodule just below dermis and are commonly seen in patients of lung or breast C_A.

Treatment

It is governed by type of malignancy as well as site and size of the lesion. Both surgery and radiotherapy field good results in majority of cases. The choice is also dictated by comparative functional and cosmetic results.

Surgery is Usually Advocated in Following Situations

i. **Malignant melanoma**–Wide excision is treatment of choice. Malignant melanomas are otherwise not considered radiosensitive to radiotherapy (RT).
ii. Few sites, e.g. hand, sole of foot because of poor vascular supply tolerate radiation poorly therefore leading to fibrosis.
While in scrotal C_A if radiotherapy is employed underlying testis will also get the radiations. Therefore in such sites surgery should be advocated.
iii. If bone is invaded surgery, will usually be required.
iv. In conditions where there are radiation failures or recurrences.
   - **Radiotherapy** can be given by brachytherapy or external radiations (both photons and electrons) depending upon the site.

> ***Note:*** *Many varieties are available in X-ray (any voltage from Grenz rays for very superficial to deep X-ray or cobalt beam for thick lesions), for brachytherapy purposes radium (or its substitutes in the form of needles or tubes) as implants or surface moulds, gold grains implants or moulds.*

   - For tumours of back of hand, forehead, chest, pinna, brachytherapy mould is preferred.

> ***Note:*** *For facial tumour particularly around eye, nose, nasolabial fold, radiotherapy employing ELECTRON BEAM is preferred.*

- **Planning technique**: Limits of skin tumour should be established by careful examination. The depth of tumour must be assessed particularly at sites such as inner canthus where deep tumour infiltration along the medial border of orbit may occur. Regional lymph nodes must be examined. Proper and optimum shielding must be done depending upon the site, e.g. lesions on eyelid when given radiotherapy treatment, eye shields incorporating thick lead are used to protect the cornea and lens.

Dose Prescription

- **Orthovoltage**: Most superficial lesions are treated with 90 KV X-rays (2 mm as HVT, 25 cm. FSD). With thicker lesion being treated with 120 KV or 150 KV electrons.

> ***Note:*** *Ideal for lesions over bone or catilage (e.g. in ear or nose).*

Dose:

Small lesion: 4000 rads (4500 R) in 9 fractions given in 3 weeks (three fractions per week) or 4000 rads in 10 fractions given in two weeks (daily fractions).

Intermediate lesion: (3 to 5 cm in favourable sites) 4500 rads (5000 R) in 15 daily fractions given in 3 weeks or 4500 rads (4800 to 5000 rads) in 12-13 fractions given in two and a half weeks.

Large lesion: Within favourable features poorly vascularized skin, e.g. lower leg, pinna, nasal cartilage) 4500 to 5000 rads (5000-5500 rads) in 20 fractions delivered in 4 weeks.

Squamous Cell C_A

- **Small lesions:** 5000 rads (5500 R) in 10 fractions given in two weeks.

- **Large lesions:** are best treated with electron or megavoltage with radiation, the doses being 6000 rads in 30 fractions over 6 weeks.

Patients Care

i. Every effort should be made to keep the skin dry and trauma must be avoided.
ii. Acute erythema may be controlled by local steroid cream.

C_A OESOPHAGUS

> ***Note:*** *The oesophagus extends from 15 to 40 cm from upper incisor tooth.*

- Early spread of cancer ensues longitudinally in submucosal tissues and lymphatics. Spread through the muscle wall occurs later, and since there is no covering, mediastinal structure involvement is very common like trachea, bronchus, various nerves.

> ***Note:*** *Simultaneously the disease may also spread by lymph nodes in mediastinum.*

Problems encountered in planning for oesophageal treatment

i. The close proximity of oesophagus to the spinal cord.
ii. Curvature of its position in thorax.
iii. Since there is a tendency for the tumour to spread along the submucosa, therefore much longer margins of apparantly normal tissue being included in the treatment volume.

Clinical Feature

Progressive dysphagia is the cardinal symptoms as the disease progresses, there can be weight loss, jaundice because of the liver involvement.

Assessment of primary disease is determined by barium swallow and esophagoscopy and diagnosis is confirmed by biopsy.

- X-ray chest, may show widening of mediastinum, any secondary in chest, or elevated diaphragm due to phrenic nerve palsy.

- CAT scan delineates the disease as well as may show involvement of mediastinal nodes.
- Treatment modalities– Surgery: Possible only in minority of cases.

  Contraindications include: Poor general condition, evidence of spread beyond oesophagus, length is > 5 cm, anaplastic growth.

ROLE OF RADIOTHERAPY

For C_A upper one-third of oesophagus radiotherapy is the treatment of choice because:

i. In upper part, histopathologically, it is squamous cell C_A, which is considered to be sensitive to radiation.
ii. **Surgery** as such is technically difficult in upper region.

For lower part or one-third of oesophagus, surgery is the treatment of choice because–

- In lower part is adenocarcinoma which is not considered to be radio-responsive.
- Surgery is easier in lower part of oesophagus.

MODE OF RADIOTHERAPY

It can be given as sole mode of treatment or can be pre- or post-operative.

Technique–Because the longitudinal and lateral extent of cancer spread is difficult to define, it is advisable to irradiate oesophagus with generous margins both in its depth as well as in length.

A. C_A upper end of oesophagus

It presents considerable problems. This is because of the "depth changes" of oesophagus from the anterior surface of patient varying with its position in the neck and thorax.

This can be solved by–

a. It is usually possible to position in supine with support behind the shoulders and neck to straighten out the cervical and upper thoracic spine, so that oesophagus presents a relatively linear horizontal volume.

b. Since there is a considerable changes in depth of oesophagus from neck to thorax associated with slope of the chest. This can be overcome by the use of a 3 field plan in which depth of the tumour. The other two fields may be postero-oblique or anterolateral wedged fields.

Field size: Supraclavicular nodes are included in the field. Generous margins of field are taken.

B. C_A lower oesophagus

It can be either a 3 field technique throughout or treating in two phases. The first phase being anterior and posterior opposing field to be followed by 3 field technique. This arrangement minimise dose to peripheral lung tissue.

However, care must be taken not to exceed tolerance dose of spinal cord (4000 to 4500 rads) during 2nd phase of treatment.

It is usual to add in upper and lower margins, 5 cm clear margins of tumour. Approximate use of wedge also improves the dose distribution. The 3 field planning can be done by using isocentric rotation or by beam directed technique like pin and arc.

Lung correction as described in C_A lung.

- **Dose:**

Phase I–4000 to 4500 rads/in 4-5 weeks to entire volume.

Phase II–Boost to reduced volume to a total dose of 6000 to 6500 R rads in 6 to 6½ weeks with lung correlation.

Precautions: Patient should be advised to take adequate fluid intake, ryles tube feeding or feeding gastrostomy is done depending upon the severity of dysphagia.

C_A PROSTATE

It is one of the leading cancer in men above 50 years of age.

Applied anatomy–Prostate gland lies between the pubic symphysis and the anterior rectal wall and is closely applied to the bladder neck and seminal vesicle. Lymphatics drain from prostate gland to pelvic nodes which finally drain into para-aortic nodes.

> **Note:** *C_A prostate metastasize most commonly to skeleton (e.g. pelvic bones, vertebrae etc). Liver, Lungs and occasionally brain may be involved by distant metastasis.*

Sign and Symptoms

a. **Early detection**: Since patient with localized prostatic C_A are usually asymptomatic, diagnosis is most often made during a routine rectal examination, however, now it can be made by US examination (Transrectal probe). There may be unsuspected C_A in a surgical specimen of prostate removed for benign prostatic hypertrophy.

b. Early symptomatic presentation may involve difficulty in starting the urinary stream, urinary bleeding, dribbling of urine and urinary retention.

c. In advanced cases, the clinical presentation may be bladder outlet obstructive symptoms with urinary retention, increased frequency, hesitancy, and narrow stream. Most patient with advanced disease present with bone pains from metastatic disease.

> **Note:** *Isolated haematuria is a very uncommon presentation.*

Pathology–Prostatic C_A are nearly always ADENOCARCINOMAS.

Grading– Grade I – Well differentiated.
Grade II – Moderately differentiated.
Grade III & IV – Poorly differentiated.

> **Note:** *The grading of carcinoma has got an important prognostic value.*

Staging–Several staging systems employed in oncological practice but the following staging is made that contains salient features of most classification.

Stage 'A' – Clinically unsuspected.
A_1 – 3 or less foci, well differentiated.

A_2 – Diffuse or more than 3 foci, poorly differentiated and more extensive than A_1.

Stage 'B' – Clinically palpable but asymptomatic prostatic nodule.

B_1 – less than 2 cm involving 1 lobe.

B_2 – greater than 2 cm, diffusely involved.

Stage 'C' – Extensive tumour with extension beyond the prostatic capsule without evidence of metastasis.

Stage 'D' – Metastatic carcinoma.

D_1 – Involvement of pelvic lymph nodes below the aortic bifurcation.

D_2 – Lymph node involvement above the aortic bifurcation and/or distant metastasis to other sites, e.g. bones, liver, etc.

ASSESSMENT OF DISEASE

i. The local extent of tumour is defined by rectal examination, cystoscopy and bimanual examination of pelvis.

> ***Note:*** *Rectal digital examination is still the best test for detecting C_A prostate.*

ii. Biochemical evaluation includes a complete blood counts, serum acid phosphatase, LDH, and serum alkaline phosphatase, LFT and renal tests.

iii. X-ray done are IVP, chest X-ray PA view, bone scan, pelvic CAT scan and lymphangiogram, transrectal USG examination.

iv. Surgical evaluation includes biopsy resection of the entire prostate gland with or without lymph nodes.

Principles of Treatment

When disease is localized either surgery or radiotherapy yield good results for cure. Hormonal manipulation is useful in palliative therapy.

- **Stage A**–Patient of stage A, prostatic CA are best treated by close follow up. They are at very low risk of developing metastasis with almost 10 years survival being 95 to 100%.

- **Stage A_1 and A_2**–Patient of stage A_2 have much more biologically aggressive form of disease and in addition about 25% of patient have metastasis to pelvic nodes. In contrast to stage A_1, stage A_2 has 5 years survival about 60%.

> ***Note:*** *Here radiotherapy is the treatment of choice. External beam radiation by megavoltage radiation to doses of 6500–7000 rads to the prostate by three field (one anterior and two posterior oblique) can effectively control local disease.*

- **Stage B**–Here two modalities surgery and radiotherapy are used. Surgery consists of radical prostatectomy. Radiotherapy can be external radiation to prostate and pelvis or interstitial implant. External radiotherapy is delivered by employing megavoltage therapy (cobalt or linear accelerator) the dose being 6500 to 7000 rads by three field or four field technique including pelvic nodes also.

  Interstitial radiation with I_2^{-125} prostatic implant has been used to treat localized prostatic C_A (stage B_1 B_2 and C). This technique should be employed as sole modality only in the absence of pelvic nodal involvement.

> ***Note:*** *In most cases combined lymphadenectomy or pelvic irradiation with an implant is employed when pelvic nodes are positive.*

- **Stage C**–All treatment modality for stage 'B' has been applied to patient with stage 'C' disease.
- **Stage D**–External radiotherapy by megavoltage equipment at a doses in the range of 5000 rads may be quite effective in the treatment of massive pelvic extension of C_A prostate or extensive lymph node involvement, which may produce pelvic pain or haematuria or by oedema because of lymphatic obstruction.

> ***Note:*** *Orchidectomy and or oestrogen may be used.*

Irradiation of Breast Prior to Hormonal Treatment

Gynaecomastia is an unwanted side effect of oestrogen treatment which is seen very commonly and may cause pain and discomfort in addition to embarrassment.

> ***Note:*** *This may be prevented by giving external radiotherapy by employing ports delivering 1200 rads midplane dose to each breast in three fractions using cobalt or 4 mv photon beam usual field size is 8 × 8 cm.*

Treatment for Painful Bony Metastasis

Painful metastasis are very common in advanced disease. They usually response to irradiation or orchidectomy. If using external radiotherapy, the painful bony metastases are treated to doses of 4500 to 5000 rads with conventional fractionation.

LYMPHOMAS

Lymphomas may be classified either Hodgkin's or non-Hodgkin's.

Hodgkin's Lymphoma

Staging-Ann-Arbor Staging

Stage I – Involvement of one nodal region.

Stage II – Involvement of two or more nodal regions on the same side of diaphragm.

Stage III – Disease limited to lymph nodes involving to both sides of diaphragm.

Stage IV – Extranodal involvement, other than spleen.

It is further subdivided into A and B, S and E.

'A'– No symptoms as defined in 'B' category.

'B'– Patients having fever more than 38°C, weight loss (over 10% of body weight in last 6 months) and night sweats.

'S'– Spleen involved pathologically.

'E'– Extension outside the lymph nodes. Staging can be clinical staging or pathological staging or both.

Investigations to be Done in Hodgkin's Lymphoma

- Thorough history taking, with attention to 'B' symptoms and careful physical examination with attention to all lymph nodes the following investigations are mandatory for the purposes of clinical staging.
- Surgical biopsy, detailed haemogram with ESR, serum chemistry, including LFT, kidney tests and radiological studies in the form of chest X-ray, IVP, lymphangiogram, skeletal survey.
- If possible CAT scan of thorax and abdomen, USG abdomen, bone marrow biopsy in patients with unexplained anaemias, stage III and IV with B symptoms with raised serum alkaline phosphatase or where X-ray or bone scan reveal any bone disease.
- Staging laparotomy is done in selected number of cases and its role is to define the extent of disease in abdomen particularly the spleen.
- With the advent of newer radiological techniques like CAT scan, USG, and MRI scan, the indication for staging laparotomy are limited and depends upon the individual decision. It has its own merits and demerits.

Treatment

The intention is to treat radically because even in stage IV, if treatment plan is judiciously made it is considered to be curable. This has been achieved owing to better diagnostic and therapeutic machines, giving sharp beams with better penetration, computer aid, better chemotherapeutic agents as well as better understanding of radiology life TDF (Split course) and biological behaviour of the disease.

> ***Note:*** *It is opined that if the disease and its contiguity can be encompassed in radiation field, radiotherapy is notwithstanding the treatment of choice.*

Radiotherapy (RT)

- Hodgkin's disease or lymphoma should be treated by MEGAVOLTAGE equipment preferably a linear accelerator so that large fields with shorter treatment times and sharp edges can be obtained.
- There should be atomized alloy block capabilities to protect normal tissues at risk, like lungs, spinal cord and (block B card after 2500 rads), larynx, lens (ask patient to look upward), head of humerus, cerebellum (2 : 1 loading) at risk are also kidneys testis and ovaries.
- The technique of treatment is very important. Fields are usually treated parallel opposed and daily doses are usually 180 to 200 rads/day to a total dose of 3600 to 4400 rads.

> ***Note:*** *Typically 3600 rads are given to clinically negaitve nodes, 4000 rads to clinically positive nodal areas and occasionally 4400 rads to areas of persistent bulky lymphadenopathy, so called boost.*

Various specific fields which have been evolved to treat nodes in one contiguous treatment volume includes:

Mantle

In general, this field includes all relevant nodes above diaphragm like cervical, supraclavicular, infraclavicular, mediastinal and hilar nodes.

> ***Note:*** *Some oncologists do waldeyering also if upper deep cervical nodes are involved.*

Mantle can be minimantle, extended mantle and inverted Y.

- Minimantle–Same as mantle without mediastinal or hilar nodes.
- Extended mantle–Mantle including para-aortic nodes to L_2 (some advocate L_3 or L_4). Advocated in cases where spleen are present because in this field area of spleen can be included and usually done in IAs, IIAs.

- Inverted 'Y': Spleen or splenic pedicle, para-aortic, iliac and femoral nodes.

  Para-aortic and splenic pedicle: Para-aortic nodes (to approximately L_4) splenic pedicle.

> ***Note:*** *These specific fields may be treated sequentially (in order to allow bone marrow recovery) and are referred to as TOTAL NODAL IRRADIATION: Mantle and Inverted* γ *(TNI)*

Subtotal nodal irradiation: Mantle and para-aortic splenic pedicle.

General Treatment Policy Adopted in Cases of Hodgkin's Disease/ Lymphoma

Stage IA, IIA : In lymphocytic predominance stage, extended mantle is sufficient and TNI is not needed. Chemotherapy (CT) not given.

> ***Note:*** *Some haematologists use TNI.*

Stage IB, IIB : Some haematologists advocate radiotherapy only as TNI. Their argument is that 'B' symptoms disappear with disappearance of disease and chemotherapy need not be added because of long-term risk of LEUKAEMIA. But if 'B' symptoms do not disappear CT can be added and disease can still be salvaged with overall excellent results. While the 2nd opinion is that in view of 'B' symptoms treat it, as advanced disease to begin with that is radiotherapy.

> ***Note:*** *TNI to be followed by chemotherapy (CT).*

Stage IIIA : Radiotherapy alone TNI is the treatment of choice. But if associated with massive mediastinal adenopathy (that is > one-third of thoracic diameter) then there are three opinions (i) split course radiotherapy, (ii) whole lung is supposed to be at risk or (iii) CT to be followed by radiotherapy.

Stage IIIB–IV – Here mainstay of treatment is CT and radiotherapy is given only for symptomatic areas, pathological fractures, compression, painful bony lesions.

Chemotherapy (CT): Two most popular regimens are advocated.

- MOPP regimen : M–Mustine hydrochloride.
  O–Oncovin.
  P–Procarbazine.
  P–Prednisolone.
- ABVD regimen : A–Adriamycin.
  B–Bleomycin.
  V–Vincristin.
  D–Dacarbazine.

RADIATION THERAPY AT A GLANCE

Introduction

Radiotherapy may annihilate neoplasia with minimal damage to nearby normal tissue thereby preserving good functional as well as cosmetic results.

> **Note:** *All human being rather all creatures are constantly exposed to natural/artificial sources of ionizing radiations. Airline travel and mining both increase exposure to background radiation.*

- Aircraft travel at 30,000 feet above see level exposes individuals to a dose equivalent of 0.5 mrem/hour.
- Radiation originating inside body comes mainly from radioactive potassium (K^+), which emits β and γ rays.
- Lungs are exposed to radiation from inhaled air, which contains small amounts of radioactive RADON.
- Cosmic exposure contributes ~28 m rem per year.
- The ground and internal sources contribute ~26 and 27 mrem/year.

> **Note:** *The most prominent man made sources of radiation include X-ray machine, nuclear arsenels and radioactive medications.*

- Equal doses of different types of radiation (X-ray, γ-ray, electron, or β-ray, proton, neutron, α-particles) do not necessarily produce equal biologic effects; thus 1 Gy of neutrons produces a greater biologic effect than 1 Gy of X-rays.

> **Note:** *In general, the biologic effects produced by a given dose of radiation can be quantified by the relative biologic effectiveness (RBE) value, which relates than to the effects produced by 250 KeV photon radiation as a standard. Thus, the greater the RBE value for a given type of radiation, the greater the biologic effect.*

- The RBE value will be greater for more densely ionizing radiation like NEUTRONS. The RBE value depends on the LET, the dose, the dose rate and the nature of the biologic system.
- The LET (Linear energy transfer) is the amount of ionizing radiation occurring per unit length of the radiation track. It is usually expressed as Kilovolts (KV) per micron and increases with the square of the change of the incident particle.

> ***Note:*** *High LET radiation differ from conventional Low LET radiation in destroying the tissues.*

- With high LET radiation, both hypoxic as well as oxygenated cells respond equally to it while with low LET radiation hypoxic cells take almost three times the doses that produce killing effects in oxygenated tissues/cells.
- Low LET radiation must produce multiple hits on DNA to destroy a cell, while high LET radiation need just a single hit on DNA to kill a cell.
- X-ray when absorbed causes ionization by 3 ways like–
  - i. Photoelectric effect.
  - ii. Compton effect, and
  - iii. Pair production.

> ***Note:*** *At low energies (30 to 100 KeV) as in diagnostic radiology, the photoelectric effect is important. The photoelectric effect varies as a function of the cube of the atomic number of the material exposed (Z^3); this fact explains why bone is visualized much better than soft tissue on radiographs.*

- At higher energies, as used in therapeutic radiology, the compton effect dominates.
- Radiation must produce double-strand breaks in DNA to kill a cell because mammalian cell has capacity to repair single strand damage.
- Radiation can also produce effects indirectly by interacting with water (H_2O) to generate free radicals, which can damage the cells.

> ***Note:*** *Free radicals are highly reactive chemical entities that lack a stable number of outer shell electrons. A free radical is not stable and has a lifespan of a fraction of a second. It is estimated that most X-ray induced cell damage is due to the formation of hydroxyl radicals, as follows:*

X-rays + $H_2O \rightarrow H_2O^+ + e^-$
$H_2O^+ + H_2O \rightarrow H_3O^+ + OH$
$OH \rightarrow$ Cell damage.
The usual end result of radiation damage is cellular death.

> ***Note:*** *Patients who receive radiation have a significant risk of neoplasm for at least two to three decades after their exposure.*

- Chromosome abnormalities typically occur in cells irradiated in the G1 phase of the cell cycle. If cells are irradiated in G2 phase then chromatid aberrations may result.

> ***Note:*** *Lymphocyte analysis may provide evidence of recent total body exposure. The minimum dose that can be detected by peripheral lymphocyte analysis is about 0.1 to 0.2 Sv (10 to 20 rem).*

- **Cell survival curve (CSC)**– represents the relationship between the dose and the fraction of surviving cell has both linear and exponential components.

> ***Note:*** *The* ***linear component*** *results from double standard chromosomal breaks produced by single hits. The exponential components represents breaks produced by multiple hits.*

- For **X-rays** or **γ-ray**, the dose response curve has a shoulder that is followed by a straight line curve as the dose is increased.

> ***Note:*** *The shoulder appears to represent the cell's ability to repair sublethal injury.*

- For α-**particles** or **lower energy neutrons**, the dose-response curve is a straight line from the origin. Thus, the survival rate is an exponential function of the dose.

> **Note:** *In all mammalian cell lines studied, increases in the RADIATION DOSE decreases the cells survival rate.*

- A number of factors may contribute to a reduced sensitivity to radiation in human tumours *in vivo*, including extrinsic factors such as HYPOXIA and INTRINSIC FACTORS such as expression of particular oncogenes including 'ras'.

> **Note:** *The BIOLOGIC BASIS of such altered sensitivity to radiation in human has not yet been fully defined.*

- Four important physiological processes that ensure after radiation exposure can be summarized as 4 'R's- viz
  i. Repair ii. Reoxygenation
  iii. Repopulation iv. Redistribution.
  i. Repair– means ability of the cell to repair itself following radiational injury. It is dependent on temperature and is thought to represent the enzymatic mechanism for healing intracellular injury.
  ii. Reoxygenation– is a process whereby O_2 and nutrients are actually better distributed to viable cells following radiation injury and cell killing.
  iii. Repopulation– the ability of the cell population to continue to divide and to replace dying and dead cell.
  iv. Redistribution that reflects the variability of a cells radiosensitivity over the cell cycle.

> **Note:** *Radiosensitivity may vary through the cell cycle by as much as a factor of '3'.*

- The G1 phase has the most variable length of all the phases of the cell cycle.
- For most cell lines, cells that have a short G_1 period are most sensitive at the G_2/mitosis interface, less sensitive in G_1 and most resistant toward the end of the synthesis(s) phase.
- Radiotherapy is effective in cancer treatment when it exerts greater cytotoxic effects on tumour cells than on normal tissues, i.e. improving the therapeutic index.

- A major determinant of the therapeutic index is exploiting differences in the four 'R's between tumour cells and normal tissues.
- **Fractionated radiation** exploits differences in the four 'R's between tumour and normal tissues, thereby improving the therapeutic index (T_1).

Normal Tissue Response to Radiation

- **Therapeutic radiation** leads to **acute effects** that ensues during treatment and resolves a few weeks after the completion of therapy. **Late effects** are also produced by radiotherapy and typically do not occur until several months or years after treatment is delivered.

> ***Note:*** *The clinical response to radiation may be related to the interaction of various growth factors and cytokines.*

As for example– Radiation may induce growth factors and cytokines such TNF and IL-1.

- Tumour necrosis factor (TNF) can induce fibroblasts proliferation and enhance the inflammatory response.
- TNF and IL-1 have been shown to radioprotect haematopoietic cells *in vitro* by increasing the D_0 of the cell survival curve.
- TNF also enhances killing of a human tumour cell line by irradiation.
- TNF may produce radioprotection or radiosensitization, depending on the cell type.

> ***Note:*** *The degree and the duration of functional recovery of normal tissues are related to the number of stem cell surviving after irradiation. If the stem cells are destroyed in the irradiated volume and replacement from adjacent tissues is inadequate, radiation injury will persists, causing late toxic effects. True late effects of radiation develop independent of early reactions; they may also occur despite recovery from acute radiation injury.*

- The clinical manifestation of irradiation will depend on the volume of the organ irradiated, the total dose, the dose per fraction, and the length of time taken to deliver the dose and probably genetic/biologic factors. Dose per fraction is the most important factor determining normal tissue effects. This is why daily fractionation doses of 180 c Gy to 200 c Gy are used in most curative treatment situations.

Therapeutic Radiation (TR)

Radiotherapy is a physical form of treatment that damages any tissue in its path. In the target tissue, radiation damages DNA (usually single-strand breaks) and generates free radicals from cell water that are capable of damaging cell membranes, proteins and organelles.

- Radiation damage is dependent on O_2.

> **Note:** *Hypoxic cells are more resistant to radiation treatment.*

So, augmentation of O_2 is the basis for radiation sensitization.

> **Note:** *Sulfhydryl compounds interfere with free radical generation and may act as radiation protectors.*

Organ	*Injury*	*Mini. TD/5/5*	*Maxi. TD/50/5*	*Whole or partial*
1. Bone marrow	Aplasia	250	450	Whole
	Pancytopenia	3000	4000	Segmental
2. Liver	Acute and	2500	4000	Whole
	Chronic hepatitis	1500	2000	Whole (strip)
3. Stomach	Perforation, ulcer, hemorrhage	4500	5500	100 cm
4. Intestine	Ulcer, perforation	4500	5500	400 cm
	Haemorrhage	5000	6500	100 cm
5. Brain	Infarction, necrosis	5000	6000	Whole
6. Spinal cord	Infarction, necrosis	4500	5500	10 cm
7. Heart	Pericarditis, Pancarditis	4500	5500	60%
8. Lung	Acute and	7000	8000	25%
	Chronic	3000	3500	100 cm
	Pneumonitis	1500	2500	Whole
9. Kidney	Acute and chronic	1500	2000	Whole (strip)
	Nephrosclerosis	2000	2500	Whole
10. Foetus	Death	200	400	Whole

- **Therapeutic radiation (TR)** is delivered in 3 ways: **Teletherapy, brachytherapy and systemic therapy**.

> ***Note:*** *The most commonly used form of RT is teletherapy.*

- X-ray and g-rays are the forms of radiation most commonly used in cancer treatment. They are both electromagnetic, nonparticulate waves that cause the ejection of an orbital electron when absorbed. This orbital electron ejection is called IONIZATION.
- X-rays are generated by linear accelerators. γ-rays are generated from decay of atomic nuclei in radioisotopes such as cobalt and radium. These waves behave biologically as pockets of energy called photons.
- Particulate forms of radiation are also used in certain circumstances. Electron beams have a very low tissue penetrance and are used to treat skin conditions like MYCOSIS FUNGOIDES.
- Neutron beams may be somewhat more effective than X-rays in treating salivary gland tumours.
- The energy of radiation determines its ability to penetrate tissue. Low energy orthovoltage beams (150 to 400 KV) scatter when they strike the body. Such beams results in more damage to adjacent normal tissues and less radiation delivered to the tumour.
- Megavoltage radiation (> 1 MeV) has very low lateral scatter; this produces a skin-sparing effect, more homogeneous distribution of the radiation energy and greater deposit of the energy in the tumour, or target volume.
- The tissues that the beam passes through to get to the tumour are called the **transit volume**.
- The maximum dose in the target volume is often the cause of complications to tissues in the transit volume, and the minimum dose in the target volume influences the likelihood of tumour recurrence.

> ***Note:*** *Dose homogeneity in the target volume is the goal.*

- Radiation is quantitated on the basis of the amount of radiation absorbed in the patient, not based upon the amount of radiation generated by the machine.
- Radiation dose is measured by placing detectors at the body surface or circulating the dose based on radiating phantoms that resembles human form and substance.
- Radiation dose has 3 determinants: (i) Total absorbed dose (ii) number of fractions, (iii) and time.
- A typical course of RT should be described as 4500 cGy delivered to a particular target (e.g. mediastinum) over 5 weeks in 180-cGy fractions.

> ***Note:*** *Most curative RT programs are delivered once a day, 5 days a week in 150 to 200 cGy fractions.*

- Although radiation may interfere with many cellular processes, many experts are of the opinion that a cell must undergo a double strand DNA break from radiation in order to be killed. The factors that influence tumour cell killing include the D_0 of the tumour (the dose required to deliver an average of one lethal hit to all the cells in a population), the D_q of the tumor (the threshold dose–a measure of the cell's ability to repair sublethal damage), hypoxia, tumour mass, growth fraction and cell cycle time and phase (cells in late G_1 and S are more resistant).

> ***Note:*** *Rate of clinical response is not predictive some cells do not die after radiation exposure until they attempt to replicate.*

- Compounds that incorporate into DNA and alter its stereochemistry (e.g. halogenated pyrimiding, cisplatin) augment radiation effects. **Hydroxyureas**, another DNA synthesis inhibitor, also potentiates radiation effects. Compound that deplete **thiols** (e.g. buthionine, sulfoximine) may also augment radiation effects.

> ***Note:*** *Hypoxia is a major factor that interfere with radiation effects.*

- Radiotherapy (Teletherapy) can be used alone or together with chemotherapy to produce cure of localized tumours and control of the primary site of disease in tumours that have disseminated.
- Radiotherapy is a component of curative treatment for a number of disease including breast C_A, Hodgkin's disease, head and neck C_A, prostate C_A and gynaecologic C_A.
- Radiotherapy can also be used to palliate disease symptoms in a variety of settings: relief of bone pain from metastatic disease, control of brain metastases, reversal of spinal cord compression and superior vena caval obstruction, shrinkage of painful masses, and opening threatened airways.

> **Note:** *In high risk settings, RT can prevent the development of leptomeningeal disease and brain metastases in acute leukemia and lung cancer.*

- **RT (Brachytherapy)** involves placing a sealed source of radiation into or adjacent to the tumour and withdrawing the radiation source after a period of time precisely calculated to deliver a chosen dose of radiation to the tumour. This approach is often used to treat brain tumours and cervical cancer.
- The difficulty with brachytherapy is the short range of radiation effects (the INVERSE SQUARE LAW) and the inability to shape the radiation to fit the target volume.

> **Note:** *Normal tissue may receive substantial exposure to the radiation, with attendant radiation enteritis or cystitis in C_AC_X or brain injury in brain tumours.*

Radionuclides and Radioimmunotherapy

> **Note:** *The radiation oncologists and nuclear medicine doctor give this treatment.*

i. I^{131} is used to treat thyroid C_A. It emits γ-rays that destroy the normal as well as thyroid C_A.

ii. Strontium (Sr^{89}) and Samarium 153 are preferentially taken up by bone particularly sites of new bone formation. Both are capable of controlling bone metastases and the pain associated with them, but the dose limiting toxicity is myelosuppression.

- Monoclonal antibodies and other ligands can be attached to radioisotopes by conjugation (for nonmetallic isotopes) and by chelation (for metallic isotopes), and the targeting moiety can result in the accumulation of the radionuclide preferentially in tumour.
- Iodine 131-labelled anti CD-20 and yttrium 90-labelled anti-CD 20 are active in B cell lymphoma, and other labelled antibodies are being evaluated. Thyroid uptake of labelled I_2 is blocked by cold iodine. Dose limiting toxicity is myelosuppression.

Photodynamic therapy

> **Note:** *Porphyrins, phthalocyanines are chemical components that are selectively taken up by cancer cells by some unknown mechanism.*

- When light, usually delivered by a LASER beam on cell containing these compounds, free radicals are generated and the targeted cells die.
- HAEMATOPORPHYRINS and LIGHT are being utilized with increased frequency to treat skin cancer, ovarian cancer, C_A lung, colon, rectum, and oesophagus.

> **Note:** *Palliation of recurrent locally advanced disease can sometimes be dramatic and last many months.*

- Bone is among the most RADIORESISTANT organs, radiation effects being manifested mainly in children through premature fusion of the epiphyseal growth plate.

> ***Note:*** *The male testis, female ovary and bone marrow are the most sensitive organs. Any bone marrow in a radiation field will be eradicated by therapeutic irradiation.*

- Heart, skeletal muscle and nerves are more resistant to radiation effects. In radiation resistant organs, the vascular endothelium is the most sensitive component.
- **Acute toxicities** include mucositis, skin erythema (ulceration in severe cases) and bone marrow toxicity. These can be alleviated by interrupting the treatment.
- Chronic toxicity includes the following and usually much more serious in nature.
  a. Radiation of head neck region cause thyroid failure.
  b. Cataracts and retinal damage can lead to blindness.
  c. Salivary glands stop making saliva, which leads to dental caries and poor dentition.
  d. Taste and smell can be affected.
  e. Mediastinal irradiation leads to a threshold increased risk of fatal myocardial infarction.
  f. Other late vascular effects include chronic constrictive pericarditis, lung fibrosis, viscus stricture, spinal cord transection and radiation enteritis.
  g. A serious late toxicity is the development of 2nd solid tumours in or adjacent to radiation fields such tumours may develop in any organ or tissue and occur at a rate of about 1% per year beginning in the 2nd decade after treatment.
  h. Some organs may vary in susceptibility to radiation carcinogenesis.
     – Women under age 30 experience a ≥ 100-fold increase in the incidence of breast C_A after chest or mantle-field radiation. Women treated after age 30 have little or no increased risk of breast C_A.

> ***Note:*** *No data suggest that a threshold dose of therapeutic radiation exists below which the incidence of 2nd cancers is decreased. High rates of 2nd tumours have been documented in people who receive as little as 1000 cGy.*

- **CNS** has been described as relatively resistant to radiation. When the human brain is treated with standard fractionation (180 to 200 cGy/day) acute reactions are seldom observed.

> ***Note:*** *Subacute CNS reactions to radiation treatment are more common. The C/M may include* ***Lhermitte's sign****, which is a self-limited paraesthesia occurring with flexion of the neck. After mantle field radiation its incidence is as high as 15%.*

- A unique late effect of cranial irradiation combined with chemotherapy called as **leucoencephalopathy** has been seen in few patients. Such reaction (a necrotizing skin) usually noted 6 to 12 months after combined treatment with methotrexate and cranial irradiation.
- Dementia and dysarthria are often observed and may progress to seizures, ataxia, or death.
- **Transverse myelitis** after radiotherapy is a spinal cord reaction similar to cerebral necrosis.

> ***Note:*** *Lhermitte's sign does not correlate with transverse myelitis.*

- **Skin** reaction can be **acute** (seen within 2 weeks) of fractionated RT) or **chronic** seen starting 6 to 12 months after irradiation. If the skin reaction is severe treatment interruption will help in such cases. The irradiated area may be hyperpigmented that fades gradually. The skin becomes thin, and hair loss may be permanent.

> ***Note:*** *Radiotherapy can induce 2nd malignancy which tend to be more aggressive than cancers arising in patient without significant radiation exposure.*

- **Heart and blood vessels** when exposed to radiation therapy there is development of CAD

(Coronary artery disease). There may be acute pericarditis and pericardial effusion may be the most common clinical menifestation of radiation induced heart disease. It is usually detected by chest X-ray and confirmed by a echocardiogram.

> **Note:** *Most patient with symptomatic radiation induced constrictive pericarditis will have received **> 40 Gy** to a large portion of the heart. The risk increases significantly with cardiac doses **> 50 Gy**.*

- Chronic cardiac charges start from 6 months to several years after irradiation. The clinical manifestation includes chronic constrictive pericarditis and endocardial fibrosis–a PANCARDITIS. The clinical signs may include dyspnoea, pain chest, venous distention, pleural effusion a paradoxical pulse.
- **Lung** may show radiation pneumonitis may appear in 3 to 6 weeks if a large region of lung is irradiated to a dose > 25 Gy. Dyspnoea and cough may be severe and debilitating. Patients with symptoms of radiation pneumonitis may respond rapidly to glucocorticoids, but it has little effect on fibrotic changes. Others include bronchodilators and O_2 therapy on support.
- **GIT**– Patient may exhibit feature of **acute** gastritis. Decreased gastric acidity is seen after 15 to 20 Gy of fractionated radiotherapy. The tolerance of the stomach to radiation is also aggravated by addition of systemic chemotherapy like 5-fluorouracil.
- The germinal centres of the bowel mucosa are in the crypts of Lieberkuhn.

> **Note:** *The epithelial lining of the small bowel is the most rapidly renewed system in the human body and is completely renewed in 3 to 6 days.*

- Within 12 to 24 hours after first dose of radiotherapy, the pathological changes are seen in bowel mucosa as dead cells.

- Most clinical manifestation of chronic changes ensues 6 months and 5 years after radiotherapy. Conservative noninvasive treatment may control GIT symptoms. A low residue ELEMENTAL DIET may be beneficial.
- **Urinary bladder** generally becomes symptomatic 3 to 6 weeks after the start of radiotherapy and symptoms usually subsides in 3 to 4 weeks after completion of RT. Patient often complains of increased frequency and dysuria. Concurrent treatment with cyclophosphamide increases the severity of the acute bladder reaction.

> **Note:** *A contracted bladder can result from doses > 60 Gy.*

- **Testes and ovaries**–Type 'B' spermatogonia are exquisitely sensitive to radiation. Sertoli cells and Leydig cells are less radiosensitive than the spermatogonia. Raised levels of FSH and LH have been observed after as little as 75 cGy. Doses as low as 10 cGy to the testicles may result in injury to the type B spermatogonia.

> **Note:** *The single dose radiotherapy required for permanent sterilization on normal human males is believed to be between 6 and 10 Gy. In normal human, sperm count recovery requires 9 to 18 months after a fractionated dose of 8 to 100 cGy.*

- The radiation dose necessary to induce ovarian failure is age dependent. A single dose of 3 to 4 Gy can induce amenorrhoea in almost all women over 40 years of age. In young women, oogenesis is much less sensitive to radiation than is spermatogenesis in men.
- **Total body irradiation**–Acute radiation exposure to whole body has been studies in humans after atomic bomb explosion in Japan and Chernobyl nuclear accident.

> **Note:** *i. At doses > 100 Gy. death usually occurs 24 to 48 hours later from neurologic and CVS failure. This is called as* ***cerebrovascular syndrome****.*
> *ii. At doses between 5 and 12 Gy death may occur in a matter of days as a result of* ***GIT syndrome****.*
> *iii. At total body doses between 2 and 8 Gy death may occur 2 to 4 weeks after exposure from bone marrow failure, the* ***haemopoietic syndrome****.*

- The $^{LD}50/60$ (the dose at which 50% of the population is dead by 60 days) is around 3.25 Gy if support is not given.
- The very young and old are more radiosensitive than middle-aged and young adults. Females in general appear to be more tolerant of radiation than males.
- At doses < 8 Gy, the patient is likely to survive with supportive care.

> **Note:** *Most people exposed to doses > 10 Gy will die from GIT syndrome. Following radiation exposure, its estimation must be made quickly because bone marrow transplantation is most effective if it is done within Ist 3 to 5 days after exposure.*

- **Radiation and cancer induction**–It has been seen that following radiation exposure some nonlethal changes in DNA sequences caused by irradiation may cause malignant transformation. Thus it is not surprising that 2nd neoplasms can be caused by exposure to ionising radiation. Throughout the history of human exposure to ionizing radiation increased rates of cancer have been noted after exposure to radiation.

> ***Note:*** *The populations studied include–*
> *i. Survivors of Atomic Bomb during World War II.*
> *ii. Radium watch-dial painters who shaped their brush tips with their tongues.*
> *iii. Patients who underwent multiple fluoroscopic examination for T.B., received spinal irradiation for ankylosing spondylitis and received breast irradiation for postpartum mastitis and others.*

- Exposure to ionizatin radiation at an earlier age appears to increase the change of developing radiation-induced carcinomas.
- **Recognised examples of radiation induced cancer includes:**

a. Radiotherapy for other malignant tumours like	→ C_A thyroid, breast, gastric. → Malanoma, lung C_A, sarcomas.
b. Neck irradiation during infancy for benign conditions	→ Thyroid C_A.
c. Cranial irradiation	→ CNS tumours.
d. Breast irradiation for postpartum mastitis	→ Breast C_A.
e. Brush licking by radium dial painters	→ Bone sarcomas.
f. Uranium mining	→ Lung C_A.
g. *In utero* exposure	→ Leukaemia.

> ***Note:*** *Till todate, a safe dose of radiation is not known, that's why it is prudent to avoid routine radiation exposure until and unless judiciously warranted.*

15

Problem Oriented Radiologic Cases Seen in Clinical Practice

You Should Know

1. In an **infant** who has been presenting with bowel obstruction. The attending pediatrician upon clinical examination order an X-ray and refer it to X-ray department. The radiologist reports a classic "duble-bubble sign" the likely diagnosis whould be→
   i. Duodenal atresia.
   ii. Annular pancreas.
   iii. Formation of band across the duodenum.
2. A patient is having seborrheic dermatitis, hepatosplenomegaly, multiple lytic lesions of skull, abdominal cramps and bilateral pulmonary infiltration, the most likely diagnosis is→ **histiocytosis 'X'**.
3. Minimum time interval between the appearance of radiographic shadow in chest X-ray after the contact with a known case of pulmonary T.B. is → **Six weeks**.
4. A **41-year-old patient** with a history of having been treated for pulmonary T.B. 10 years back presents with weight loss and recurrent haemoptysis of 6 months duration. His sputum for AFB is repeatedly negative. His X-ray chest reveal a cavitatory lesion in the right upper lobe with an ill-defined opacity within it. The most appropriate line of management will be → Surgical resection.
5. **Rustam**, a 17-year-old boy with thalassemia major has been admitted with a history of fever

and respiratory distress of 10 days duration. His respiratory rate is 36 per minute arterial PO_2 is 40 mmHg and PCO_2 is 30 mm Hg. His chest X-ray shows bilateral basal infiltration. The most likely diagnosis is → **Mycoplasma pneumonia**.

6. **Mano Mian**, a 45-year-old male, who is known to be HIV positive, has been admitted with a history of fever, headache, vomiting, and drowsiness for the past seven days. The investigations to be done here to settle **aetiological diagnosis** includes–
   i. CAT scan of head.
   ii. CSF serology.
   iii. India ink preparation of CSF.
7. **Kariman**, a patient has developed sudden attack of high fever, rigor, cough and foul-smelling sputum of 3 weeks duration. On examination there is dullness with bronchial breath sounds in the above areas. Skiagram of chest shows a rounded opacity in midzone without fluid level. The most likely diagnosis here is→ **Necrotizing pneumonitis**.
8. **Kharush Mian**, a 36-year-old male with a history of renal calculi is seen because of polyuria and polydipsia. Urine examination reveals sp. gr. of 1008 and calcium oxalate crystals on microscopic examination. X-ray of KUB region reveals nephrocalcinosis. The most likely diagnosis is → HYPERPARATHYROIDISM.
9. **Genda Singh**, a 36-year-old patient who has high fever, tachycardia, haemoptysis and a lobar consolidation on chest X-ray (P.A. view) has been suffering from → **Lobar pneumonia**.
10. **Saloni**, a young lady presented with dyspnoea and tachypnoea, and treated for trauma, shock and sepsis, on examination there is arterial hypoxaemia, and diffuse alveolar and interstitial infiltrates on X-ray chest (PA view). The most likely aetiology is **adult respiratory distress syndrome**.

11. Absent stomach bubble on antenatal ultrasonography in a 32-year-old **Kulsum Bibi** is an important finding for antenatal diagnosis of → Oesophageal atresia in the foetus.
12. A **newborn** is brought with history suggesting intestinal obstruction. An upright X-ray of the abdomen shows multiple air fluid levels with areas of calcification. The most likely diagnosis is → **Meconium plug syndrome**.
13. A **4-week-old infant** has constipation and recurrent vomiting is brought to the paediatric OPD/emergency for evaluation. The attending doctor has sent this child to USG to be done. The USG of abdomen reveals dine-shaped pyloric sphincters. The most likely diagnosis is **Hypertrophic obstructive pyloric stenosis**.
14. A **9-month-old child** has two episodes of cystitis. The investigations to be done under evaluation of this child include:
    i. USG (ultrasonography).
    ii. Urine culture.
    iii. Urine sugar.
15. An **one-month-old female child** has a swelling over the back in the sacral region. There is no cough impulse in the swelling. X-ray examination shows erosion of the coccyx. The most likely clinical diagnosis would be **sacrococcygeal teratoma**.
16. In a **20-year-old Zara** has been admitted for pain abdomen off and on. An ultrasound examination shows dilated intrahepatic biliary chennels with a small gallbladder. The most likely possiblility is **common bile duct stone**.
17. **Suresh a 33-year-old alcoholics** has reported to SOPD/ emergency for pain abdomen. The attending surgeon has order postosplenogram to be done on which "pruned tree appearance" is revealed. The suggestive likely diagnosis is **cirrhosis of liver**.
18. **Rahim, a 29-year-old patient**, was diagnosed to be a case of surgical (obstructive) jaundice.

The attending surgeon has order an ultrasound to confirm the clinical diagnosis. The most suggestive USG finding is **parallel shotgun appearance**.

19. In a **22-year-old Fahim** an ultrasound of liver shows a focal lesion. The next line of investigation to confirm the diagnosis is **CAT scan**.
20. A **42-year-old Zagreb** was suspected to be a case of retroperitoneal tumour. The plain X-ray likely to reveal obliteration of psoas shadow in case of **retroperitoneal tumour**.
21. **Neha, a 6-month-old infant** has been suffering from fever, irritability and swelling of jaw for the last 3 months. The mandible is thickened and of increase density. There is a thin shell of periosteal reaction along the inferior surface. The most likely diagnosis is **infantile cortical hyperostosis**.
22. **Moin Khan, a 4½-year-old male child** has symptoms of bouts of diarrhoea and dyspnoea since 1 year. X-ray chest (PA view) reveal trachea and mediastinum shifted towards right side. Whole of the left chest is full of gas shadow's lying posteriorly. The most likely diagnosis is → **Congenital diaphragmatic hernia**.
23. **Rekha, a 49-year-old female** was admitted with fever and urinary tract disorder, odynophagia and substernal burning. Oesophagogram revealed irregular oesophageal margins with multiple shadow projections in distal half of oesophagus with totally aperistaltic distal third of oesophagus. The most likely underlying cause is **oesophageal moniliasis**.
24. **Kutty Poin, an 18-year-old female** got a routine chest radiography revealed slight rotation of heart and a large air fluid level under the dome of right diaphragm. Oral cholecystogram showed normal situated gallbladder and liver. Barium meal shows stomach on the right side. The most likely reason is **gastric hetrotaxia**.

25. A **youngman** named **Kalimullah**, complained of generalized diffused abdominal pain of burning and cramping character. Sometime getting worse after meal for last one and half year. Haemoglobin is 6 gm%. Barium meal study showed oedematous, thickened and dilated jejunal mucosal folds with segmentation of barium. These could be due to **malabsorption syndrome secondary to hookworm disease**.
26. **Nochini, a 41-year-old female** complained of pain in right lower abdomen, loss of weight and low grade fever. A tenderness was palpable in right iliac fossa. X-ray chest was normal. Barium meal shows pulling up of terminal ileum, skipping of the caecum and ascending colon with loss of normal ileocaecal angle. The most likely diagnosis is **Ileo-caecal tuberculosis**.
27. A **2-day-old infant** having bile stained vomiting with progressive abdominal distension. No meconium was passed. Anteroposterior supine and lateral views of abdomen reveal a markedly dilated caecum, transverse colon with large bowel dilatation down to sigmoid region. A barium enema study reveal complete obstruction to the flow of barium in sigmoid colon. The most likely diagnosis is **congenital atresia of sigmoid colon**.
28. **Acchan, a 38-year-old** complains of fever, right upper quadrant pain abdomen. Pain increases on deep respiration. Posteroanterior view of chest and upper abdomen reveal irregular superior border of right dome of diaphragm. Right dome of diaphragm is higher in position. Right costophrenic angle is obliterated. Air fluid level is seen in the liver. From the above C/P, it is a case of **amoebic liver abscess**.
29. **Raju, a 14-month-old male child** has been suffering from pain abdomen, dysuria and dribbling of urine. Plane X-ray shows no radio opaque calculus in KUB region. An IVP is order that

reveal clubbing of calyces on both sides, both ureters dilated. Urinary bladder exhibits irregular margin. The most likely diagnosis is **posterior urethral valve**.

30. **Jagat Mian, a 33-year-old male** complains of mild right lumbar abdominal pain, haematuria and pyuria for the last 3 years. B.P. 190/120 mm Hg. IVP shows right kidney smaller in size. Hydronephrotic changes are visible in right kidney. Right ureter is dilated. Left kidney shows normal function. The most likely diagnosis is congenital hypoplastic kidney with **chronic pyelonephritis**.
31. **Roshini, a 42-year-old lady** complains of heaviness in right renal angle with mild renal pain for the last one year. Plain X-ray shows right kidney is lower than the left. Size and shape seems to be normal position of right kidney changes more than 1½ inch in erect and supine. Right ureter is tortuous. Left kidney is normal the most likely diagnosis is **mobile kidney.**
32. **Lanrmur, a 9-year-old male** child complains of incontinence of urine since birth. Plain X-ray abdomen shows widened pubic symphisis. IVP shows mild hydro-nephrotic changes in pelvi-calyceal pattern. Urinary bladder is smaller in size. Micturating cystogram shows bilateral ureteric reflux. The most likely pathology is → **Ectopia vesicae**.
33. **Kelovia, a 55-year-old female** complains of haematuria, fever and pain in the right renal angle for the last 2 years. Right kidney is ballotable. Plain X-ray shows tissue mass shadow in right lumbar region. IVP shows delayed excretion from the right kidney. Right calyces are stretched and displaced anteriorly. No destruction or obliteration of calyces is seen. These above pathoclinicologic findings seen in cases of → **PYONEPHROSIS**.

34. **Lauruhar Pain Tonk, a 61-year-old lady** complains of pain in the left side of abdomen with a palpable mass and loss of weight for the last two years. Plain X-ray shows large left kidney. IVP reveals distortion, displacement and destruction of superior calyces by a large mass in the upper pole of left kidney. The most likely diagnosis here is → **Hypernephroma**.
35. **Nand Kishore, a 61-year-old Hindu male**, complains of recurrent attack of painless haematuria for the last 3 months. Urine examination shows red cells in plenty. IVP reveals normal functioning both the kidneys. Irregular filling defect is seen in left side of bladder and base of bladder. The most likely reason here is **C_A urinary bladder**.
36. **Bulaki Mian, a 63-year-old man** complains of dysuria; urinalysis showed no glycosuria. Blood sugar is within normal limits urine culture shows *E. coli* growth. Plain X-ray KUB region showed a big vesical and interstitial gas in the wall of urinary bladder. IVP showed changes of chronic infection pelvicalyceal pattern. The most likely diagnosis is **cystitis emphysematosa**.
37. **Rinki, a 9-year-old girl** child complains of haematuria and pain in the left side of abdomen due to blunt injury occurred 7 days back. IVP shows spill of contrast media from middle and inferior calyces of left kidney. These could be due to → **Renal injury**.
38. **Rajesh Johni, a 55-year-old male** complains of mass in the left upper abdomen for the last 2½ years. Plain X-ray shows homogenous density seen in left side of abdomen. IVP shows ectopic left kidney due to soft tissue mass displacing it downward. Left ureter is tortuous. The most likely cause is **suprarenal mass.**
39. **Fuddi Mian, a 51-year-old male** complains of frequency of micturition hesitancy, nocturia

for the last 6 months. Plain abdomen reveals no calculus. IVP shows bilateral sacculation of both sides calyces, dilated ureters both sides and filling defect in the bladder. He most likely suffers from **benign hypertrophy of prostate gland**.

40. If the **biological half-life** of a particular isotope is 3 days and the **effective half-life** is 2 days. What is the **physical half-life**?
Ans.: Six days.
41. In a **WIPE TEST** performed on all radioactive sealed sources, the wipes sample must contain the following activity to make the radioactive unit safe is less than 0.005 μci.
42. **Gamma ray spectrometer** can be made to accept in many cases only the energies selected by the operator, and reject the scattered radiation. This selective process depends on the higher the primary the better the separation.
43. A **child named Tunna** showing widened, "Box-car" shaped metacarpals prominently decalcified with lack of pneumatization of the maxillary sinuses probably suffers from **HURLER'S disease**.
44. A well-defined cystic area of smudgy rarefaction densely outlined, involving both epiphyseal and metaphyseal regions of the distal femur of an **adolescent** probably is CHONDROBLASTOMA.
45. A round, homogeneous area of destruction sharply outlined by a dense rim of bone at the distal end of a distal phalanx probably is **epithelial inclusion or epidermoid cyst**.
46. **Guddu, a 4-year-old child** showing diffuse lytic changes in both femora with periosteal elevation should have further investigation of abdomen.
47. A **well-defined pelvic mass** showing amorphous calcification and loculated destruction of the sacrum may be a chondrosarcoma but this should also be strongly considered CHORDOMA.

48. An eccentric, well-circumscribed, oval cystic lesion in the metaphyseal region of the proximal humerus shows fine, **"Egg-shell"** ballooning externally and a honeycomb appearance of fine, incomplete septa internally indicate probable → **ANEURYSMAL BONE CYST**.
49. A **well-defined bony prominence** at the anteromedial surface of the distal humerus is associated with median nerve neuralgia and represents → Supracondyloid process.
50. **Films of an otherwise healthy young adult** showing extensive, mottled cortical and medullary destruction of the distal femoral shaft suggest probably → Reticulum cell sarcoma.
51. A **6-year-old showing generally demineralized bones** with fine, linear periosteal reaction along the long bones and metaphyseal bands of radiance probably suffers from → LEUKAEMIA.
52. In **Supracondylar fractures of the humerus in children**. The distal fragment usually is displaced → Posteriorly.
53. **Manish, a 4-year-old child** showing failure to grow, anaemia, and a wooly **"MOTH EATEN APPEARANCE"** of the long bone metaphyses and skull with widened epiphyseal lines probably suffers from → **RENAL RICKETS**.
54. **Kamlesh, a 2½-year-old child** showing symmetrical cortical thickening of long bones as well as prominent muscular weakness probably has → **ENGELMANN'S disease**.
55. The **long bones of a newborn infant** show increased prominence and density of the transverse lines of calcified cartilage indicating probably → has **CONGENITAL SYPHILIS**.
56. **Painful calcification of the intervertebral disease** in the cervical spine of children has been described and indicates → a transient entity with complete regression.

57. The **cervical spine of a young 22-year-old adult** showing several fused small joints bilaterally with underdeveloped vertebral bodies sharing narrowed intervertebral discs indicates probable **childhood Still's (rheumatoid) disease**.
58. In **10-year-old Mukta,** the anteroposterior view of a hip showing widened, irregular epiphyseal line, decalcified femoral head with sharply defined epiphyseal plate of the head indicates probable → **Slipped femoral capital epiphysis**.
59. In **a patient,** a prominent and sharply demarcated pulmonary artery segment and a distinct left ventricular contour in a PA chest roentgenogram strongly suggests → **congenital absence of the pericardium**.
60. On serial chest radiograph a nodule with a **"Tumour doubling time"** of over one year increases the probability that the lesion is → **Benign tumour**.
61. A **patient named Fulki** has presented with alveolar capillary block usually manifest on chest roentgenogram as → **Diffuse disease**.
62. The finding of an "AIR ESOPHAGOGRAM" on plain roentgenograms should suggest the diagnosis of → **Systemic sclerosis**.
63. In **a right sided aortic arch**, defects of both theright and posterior aspects of the barium filled oesophagus are found when there is an aortic diverticulum on the descending portion of the aorta on the left.
64. **Bilateral stippled calcification of normal size** and shaped **adrenal in the neonate** followed by wasting and rapid death clinically is found in → **WOLMAN'S disease**.
65. When the diagnosis of **Neuroblastoma in children** is initially made, radiographically demonstrable distant metastases are present in about **68% of cases**.

66. A patient was brought to emergency for a trauma to the kidneys, **Angiography** adds little if excretory urography reveals normal appearance of the urinary tract.
67. **Maula**, a patient with metastatic thyroid carcinoma is a candidate for radioactive iodine treatment. The uptake of $^{131}I_2$ in the metastases is best enhanced by doing → **Total thyroidectomy**.
68. A pattern of **lung scan** of peripheral pulmonary hypoperfusion with circumferential zones of decreased radioactivity frequently recognized around the interlobar fissures represent → microemboli lodging in the small axial arteries of the lung periphery.
69. With the **Radioisotopic cisternographic** picture in a person of no intraventricular penetration of the tracer and large amount of radioactivity in the dilated cisterns around the brain. The diagnosis is probably **Hydrocephalus ex Vacuo**.
70. With the **patient lying** so that the median plane is parallel with the table top and the inter-pupillary line perpendicular to the film. The view to be taken is the **lateral skull**.
71. With the patient in the **supine position**, the radiographic base line is placed parallel to film is the **submentovertical position**.

16

Most Common in Radiology, Radiotherapy and Oncology

You Should Know

1. **Adrenal gland enlargement** is best diagnosed by **CAT scan**.
2. The most characteristic **"onion-peel appearance"** on X-ray is seen in **Ewing's tumour**.
3. **Myodil** is most commonly used for **myelography**.
4. Most commonly **soft tissue mamography** is used as screening test for diagnosing **early breast carcinoma (C_A)**.
5. Most commonly **dead bone** on X-ray appears as **more radio-opaque**.
6. Most commonly **subphrenic abscess** is diagnosed by **fluoroscopy**.
7. **Bronchiectasis** is most commonly diagnosed by **Bronchogram**.
8. **Aneurysm of abdominal aorta** is most commonly diagnosed by **USG** (ultrasonography).
9. X-ray skull most characteristically shows **"hair on end" appearance** in **thalassaemia major**.
10. The investigation most useful in distinguishing a renal cyst from a renal C_A is **renal arteriogram**.
11. The best test for diagnosis of **vesical rupture** after pelvic trauma is **cystogram**.
12. The most useful diagnostic aid in **trophoblastic tumour** is **USG**.
13. **"Notching of the ribs"** on X-ray, is a most characteristic feature in cases of **coarctation of aorta**.

14. **"Ulcer crater"** on barium X-ray examination mostly indicates the diagnosis of **duodenal ulcer**.
15. **"Barium enema"** is a most diagnostic procedure in cases of colon disease.
16. Most commonly **"Pipe stem appearance"** on X-ray is seen in cases of **ulcerative colitis**.
17. Radiologically **increased ICP** in adults is mostly diagnosed by **erosion of sella turcica**.
18. Most commonly **unilateral elevation of diaphragm** is due to **Scoliosis**.
19. In **urinary schistosomiasis, calcification** is most commonly seen in **urinary bladder**.
20. Mostly **early mucosal cancers of the stomach** can better be made out by **double contrast meal studies**.
21. Mostly **xeroradiography** is useful for detecting **early cancer of breast**.
22. The **earliest radiological changes in rickets** are narrowing or absence of the normal zone of provisional calcification.
23. **Left atrial enlargement** can best be made out by right anterior oblique with barium.
24. **Cerebral angiography** is most useful in demonstrating lesions of cerebral blood vessels and intracranial tumours.
25. A most **pathognomonic X-ray sign of chronic pancreatitis** is pancreatic calcification.
26. The most reliable method of diagnosis of pulmonary embolism is by **Angiography**.
27. Calcification of ascending aorta is most commonly caused by **syphilis or lues**.
28. The best view to detect the minimum pleural effusion in X-rays is **lateral view**.
29. The most common **radioisotope** used in **placental localisation** is **Iodine-132**.
30. Most commonly **radioactive iodine uptake** by thyroid is increased in cases of **thyrotoxicosis**.
31. In **thyrotoxicosis,** thyroid scarring most commonly done by using isotope-**I_2-131**.

32. The radioisotope used most commonly in liver scan is **Technetium 99**.
33. Most commonly **radioactive mould** is used in cases of **C_A penis**.
34. **Radiotherapy** is mostly curable in **Ewing's tumour**.
35. In **radiotherapy,** the most common radiation used is **gamma (γ)** rays.
36. **Postoperative radiation** is mostly useful in **Wilms' tumour**.
37. The five year survival rate is highest in **papillary C_A thyroid**.
38. The most radiosensitive tissue in human is bone marrow.
39. The most highly **radioresistant tumour** is FIBROSARCOMA.
40. The **poorest prognosis** in terms of five-year survival is offered by C_A gallbladder.
41. Most commonly **afterload intracavitory radiation** is used in carcinoma cervix (C_A C_X).
42. Most commonly **craniospinal irradiation** is indicated in acute lymphatic leukemia (ALL) after remission.
43. Most **seminoma of the testis** is highly sensitive to radiation.
44. Probably the **most sensitive cell** in the human body to **radiation** is LYMPHOCYTE.
45. Most commonly response to radiation therapy (RT) is better in ANAPLASTIC CARCINOMA.
46. Treatment by RT is most frequently indicated in C_AC_X.
47. Most pathognomonic X-ray sign of chronic pancreatitis is **pancreatic calcification**.
48. Most common **"Figure of 8"** heart is usually seen in X-ray chest in total anomalous pulmonary venous drainage.
49. Most common endocrine disorder diagnosed by X-ray of hand is **acromegaly**.

50. **Plaques of disseminated sclerosis** is best detected by MRI.
51. Unilateral hypertranslucent hemithorax on chest X-ray is seen mainly in **poliomyelitis**.
52. Sign most suggestive of C_A lung on chest X-ray is **rib erosion**.
53. For small pneumothorax, X-ray is done mostly in, expiration (PA view).
54. Most common **noninvasive diagnostic test** for **pulmonary embolism** is ventilation perfusion lung scan.
55. Best investigative procedure for **cardiac tamponade** is 2 D echocardiography.
56. Presence of calcification in an **intracranial lesion** is best made out by **CAT scan**.
57. In skull X-ray, most common cause of intracerebral calcified shadow is **oligodendroglioma**.
58. **"Bat wing appearance"** in X-ray is seen most commonly in cardiogenic pulmonary oedema.
59. **Soldier helmet skull** with deafness is most characteristic of ACROMEGALY.
60. Most commonly **fresh intracranial haemorrhage** in CAT scan appears as HYPODENSE area.
61. Most common cause of **unilateral increase in translucency** of lung field in X-ray chest PA view is rotation of patient.
62. **Oat cell C_A** most commonly metastases to bones.
63. Most commonly **honey-comb liver** is seen in ACTINOMYCOSIS.
64. **Free air under the dome of diaphragm** most commonly suggests perforation of hollow viscus.
65. Earliest radiological change in ulcerative colitis is observed in **sigmoid colon**.
66. Most commonly MAMMOGRAPHY is **high KV and low mamp technique**.
67. Density of a tissue on CAT scan is mostly measured in **Hounsfeld unit**.

68. "ACOUSTIC SHADOW" on ultrasonography (USG) is mostly due to **reflection**.
69. NMR/MRI scan is mostly based on **magnetic moment of the nucleus.**
70. Most sensitive investigation of pancreatic C_A is **angiography**.
71. Most common type of radiation used in radiotherapy is **ionizing radiation.**
72. Investigation of choice in peptic ulcer perforation is **X-ray abdomen**.
73. Investigation of choice in common bile duct stricture is **ultrasound**.
74. **Isotope renogram** most commonly reveal graphic representation of radioactivity of kidneys.
75. Most commonly postoperative radiotherapy in breast is given to prevent its recurrence.
76. Most commonly calcifying epithelioma is seen in **Pyogenic granuloma**.
77. Most commonly **"Pruned tree appearance"** on portosplenorenogram is suggestive of cirrhosis.
78. **"String sign of Kantor"** and perianal fistula are most common feature of regional enteritis.
79. **"parallel shotgun appearance"** on ultrasound is seen mostly in obstructive jaundice.
80. Most commonly radiations in X-ray are produced from electron.
81. **"Obliteration of psoas shadow"** most commonly on plain X-ray is seen in retroperitoneal tumour.
82. Investigation of choice in aortic dissection is **Transoesophageal echocardiography**.
83. Best investigation for diagnosis of postoperative biliary fistula is ERCP.
84. VUR (vesicoureteric reflux) is best demonstrated by **micturating cystourethrogram**.
85. Most commonly ischemic myocardium is distinguished from non-ischemic myocardium by **Thallium scan**.

86. Most commonly marked enlargement of left atrium occurs in **Mitral regurgitation**.
87. **"Reverse 3" deformity** of oesophagus is seen most commonly in COA (Coarctation of aorta).
88. **"Egg shell calcification"** of hilar lymph nodes is most often due to SILICOSIS.
89. Most common **cavitating lung C_A** is squamous cell C_A.
90. **"Reversed batwing" appearance** on chest X-ray is seen in **Loeffler's syndrome**.
91. Most commonly **bilateral elevation of diaphragm** is seen in ascites.
92. Most sensitive method of diagnosis of secondaries in liver is CT-guided biopsy.
93. Most commonly **"Multiple calcification"** is noted in chest X-ray in a patient following chickenpox.
94. **"SILHOUETTE Sign"** (loss of normal right heart contour on chest X-ray) most commonly associated with diseases of the right upper lobe.
95. **"Photonegative pulmonary oedema"** pattern with central sparing on chest X-ray is seen most commonly in chronic eosinophilic pneumonia.
96. **"Oligaemic lung field"** are seen most commonly in Fallot's tetralogy.
97. Best investigation to distinguish cardiac dilatation from pericardial effusion is **echocardiography**.
98. **"Calcification of diaphragmatic pleura"** is most characteristic of pneumoconiosis due to ASBESTOSIS.
99. Most accurate assessment of spleen size can be done by **colloid scan**.
100. Most sensitive investigation for detecting **minimal ascites** in USG.
101. **Ultrasound** most commonly discriminate between **solid** masses and **cystic** lesion.
102. **Tufting and mushrooming of terminal phalanges** is most characteristically seen in ACROMEGALY.

103. Investigation of choice for the diagnosis of **phaeochromocytoma** is CAT scan.
104. Most sensitive investigation for diagnosis of **demyelinating disease** is MRI/NMR scan.
105. **Mitral valve prolapse** is best diagnosed by 2D echography.
106. Best investigation for diagnosis of **pericardial effusion** is echocardiography.
107. **"Moving ball"** in lungs is seen mostly in **Aspergillosis**.
108. Most commonly **opaque hemithorax** is seen in hypoplasia lungs.
109. Calcification of pleura is seen most commonly in **haemothorax**.
110. **Multiple cysts in lungs** (Pneumatocoeles) are most commonly seen in staphylococcal infection.
111. Most common organs visualized on plain X-ray abdomen is **liver, spleen and kidney**.
112. **Osteolytic bone lesions, exophthalmos and diabetes insipidus** are most commonly seen in Hand-Schuller-Christian disease.
113. Most useful investigation in patient with jaundice is percutaneous transhepatic cholangiography.
114. **"Snowman" appearance in chest X-ray** is most diagnostic of TAPVD.
115. **M-mode echocardiography** is most diagnostic in pericardial effusion.
116. Investigation of choice for minimal bronchiectasis is bronchography.
117. Investigation of choice for detecting parathyroid pathology is **Technetium-Thallium subtraction scan**.
118. **Subperiosteal erosion** most commonly seen in hyperparathyroidism.
119. Best diagnostic method for bronchiectasis is **bronchography**.
120. **Subcutaneous calcifications** are most commonly seen in hyperparathyroidism.

121. Most common cause of **oesteoblastic pulmonary metastasis** is squamous cell C_A.
122. Mostly **air bronchogram** is seen in consolidated lungs.
123. Mostly **nephrogram** phase of IVP occurs because of dye present in collecting tubules.
124. **Pneumothorax** is best demonstrated by taking a radiograph, with the patient in end expiration.
125. Mostly **deleterious effect of ultrasound** on small organism ensues because of CAVITATION.
126. Most **radiosensitive lung cancer** is **small cell** C_A.

17 Last Moment Revision in Radiology, Radiotherapy and Oncology

You Should Know

1. The correct sequence of **cell cycle** is **G_0-G_1-S-G_2-M**.
2. High resolution CT of the chest is the ideal modality for evaluating **interstitial lung disease**.
3. **"Bone erosions"** is a recognised X-ray feature of **rheumatoid arthritis**.
4. A 55-year-old man who has been on bed-rest for the past 10 days, complains of breathlessness and chest pain. The X-ray chest (PA view) is normal. The most likely diagnosis is pulmonary thrombo-embolism and so the chief diagnostic procedure here is to do a **lung-ventilation perfusion scan**.
5. Cardiac output measured by **thermodilution technique** is unreliable in tricuspid regurgitation, low cardiac output and pulmonary regurgitation but not in VSD.
6. **"Fraying and cupping"** of metaphysis of long bones in an child does not occur in lead poisoning.
7. **"Fraying and cupping"** of **metaphysis** seen in—Rickets, hypophosphatemia/hypophosphatasia, chronic stress, copper deficiency, metaphyseal dysplasia.
8. **CT scan of a patient** with history of injury shows a biconvex hyperdense lesion displacing the grey-white matter interface. The most likely diagnosis is **extradural haemorrhage**.

9. **MRI scanning** is the best choice for evaluating a posterior fossa tumour radiologically.
10. Most suitable **radioisotope of iodine** for treating hyperthyroidism is $\mathbf{I^{131}}$.
11. **Eosinophilic granuloma** (Histiocytosis) is the most common cause in children of vertebra plana, which is characterized by remarkable flattening of vertebral body while posterior elements and disc spaces remain intact.
12. **Differential diagnosis of solitary collapsed vertebra** includes–
    - Neoplasia
        a. Metastatic (Breast, bronchus, prostate, kidney and thyroid).
        b. Multiple myeloma/plasmacytoma.
    - Osteoporosis.
    - Paget's disease.
    - Infection (Tuberculous).
    - Histiocytosis.
    - Benign tumours–Haemangioma, osteoclastoma and aneurysmal bone cyst.
    - Traumatic injury.
13. **Radioisotope cobalt 60** is commonly used as a source for external beam radiotherapy in the treatment of cancer patients.
14. **High resolution CT** of the **lung** is a specialized CT technique for greater detail of lung parenchyma and it utilizes bone algorithm for image reconstruction.
15. A **dense persistent nephrogram** may be seen in dehydration, acute ureteral obstruction and severe hydronephrosis, acute hypotension, multiple myeloma, amyloid nephropathy, urate nephropathy, renal vein thrombosis, AGN and PN, acute papillary necrosis.
16. **MIBG scan** is most sensitive for evaluating extra-adrenal **phaeochromocytoma**.
17. X-rays are produced when electron beam strikes the anode.
18. **Cysteine stones** are **radio-opaque** stones.

19. Xanthine, orotic acid, urate (allopurinol induced xanthine stones) cause **radiolucent** stones.
20. **PET** appears to be a more sensitive method than traditional imaging with CT scaning for detecting local and distant metastases in patient with non-small cell lung C_A.
21. Mostly **maximum permissible radiation** dose in **pregnancy** is **0.5 rad**.
22. **MRI rooms** are shielded completely by a continuous sheet or wire mesh of Cu^{++} or Al^{++} to shield the imager from external electromagnetic radiations, etc. It is called **Faraday cage**.
23. A patient is suspected to have **vestibular schwannoma**. The investigation of choice for its diagnosis is—Gadolinium enhanced MRI.

> ***Note:*** *It is a case of* ***acoustic neuroma*** *so gadolinium DTPA in MRI provides better visualization of tumour.*

24. **Radiological signs of scurvy** include–
    - Pelican spur.
    - Zone of demarcation near epiphysis (Wimberger sign).
    - White line of Frenkel.

> ***Note: "Soap bubble appearance"*** *is characteristically seen in* ***Giant cell tumour****.*

25. On radiography widened 'C' loop with irregular mucosal pattern on upper gastrointestinal barium series is most likely due to **carcinoma head of pancreas**.
26. **Barium study of acute pancreatitis** reveal thickening and effacement of mucosal fold, Frostberg's sign and widening or narrowing of duodenum 'C' loop. While chronic pancreatitis shows double contour and strictures.
27. **Barium study in duodenal ileus** shows widened duodenal loop with regular mucosal pattern.
28. The most penetrating beam is **gamma (γ)** rays or photons. The photons with **more energy** (18 MV) is **more penetrating** than 8 MV photons.

29. The **radiation tolerance of liver** as a whole is **40 Gy** or **4000 rads.**

> ***Note: Radiation tolerance of whole organ*** *are as follows–*
> - *Foetus – 400 rads*
> - *Bone marrow – 450 rads*
> - *Brain – 6000 rads*
> - *Kidney (whole strip) – 2000 rads*
> - *Kidney (whole organ) – 2500 rads*
> - *Liver (whole strip) – 2000 rads*
> - *Lung (whole) – 2000 rads*

30. In **gastric C_A** postoperative radiotherapy is minimally used for pain relief, etc.
31. **Postoperative radiotherapy** is used as adjuvant therapy in head and neck C_A, colonic C_A and soft tissue sarcomas.
32. **CAT scan** findings of **acute pancreatitis** include–
    - Ill defined outlines of pancreas (due to oedema).
    - Enlargement of pancreas.
    - Poor contrast enhancement (due to fat necrosis).

> ***Note:*** *Dilatation and beading of main pancreatic duct and its branches with calcification seen as beaded/string of pearls/chain of lakes and rat tail appearance on ERCP is pathognomonic of* ***chronic pancreatitis****.*

33. The **classic CAT scan** appearance of an acute subdural haematoma is crescent-shaped hyperdense lesion.

> ***Note:*** *The* ***classic CAT scan*** *picture of subacute/chronic subdural haematoma is crescent-shaped isodense/hypodense lesion respectively.*

34. The **classic CAT scan** picture of epidural haematoma in acute cases is lenticular and hyperdense while in chronic cases is lenticular and hypodense.

35. The **investigation of 1st choice** in a patient with suspected **SAH** (subarachnoid haemorrhage) should be non-contrast CAT scan.
36. **Radioisotopes** are used in mass spectroscopy, RIA and sequencing of nucleic acid.

> ***Note: ELISA*** *as it stands for enzyme linked immunoabsorbent test/assay, is based on enzymatic colour changes in evaluating the sample to be tested not using radioisotopes.*

37. The **dose of radiotherapy** recommended for pain relief in bone metastases is usually 30 Gy in ten fraction but it can also be given as 8 Gy in just single shot or fraction.
38. A patient with **cancer** received extreme degree of radiation toxicity. Further history revealed that the dose adjustment of a particular drug was missed during RT is order to prevent radiation toxicity is DACTINOMYCIN.

> ***Note:*** *Other drugs required dose adjustment includes Doxorubicin, 5–FU, Methotrexate, Bleomycin, Nitrosoureas and Etopside, etc.*

39. The **gold standard** for the **diagnosis of osteoporosis** is **dual energy X-ray absorptiometry (DEXA).**
40. **Angiographically**, the typical "beaded" or pile of plates appearance involving the internal carotid artery is observed in **Fibromuscular dysplasia (FMD)**.

> ***Note: FMD*** *affects right renal artery mainly as stenosis. Although affects the entire 3 coats (intima, media and adventitia) it is the tunica media that suffers mostly in 75% of cases. This typical C/P angiographically is due to alternating stenosis or aneurysmal lesions. Treatment is angioplasty. The other arteries involved due to FMD is iliac artery, splanchnic artery or internal carotid A.*

41. After contrast medial injection in the radiology department, a patient develops severe hypo-

tension, bronchospasm and cyanosis. This patient should be given immediately **ADRENALINE**.

> ***Note:*** *Severe reactions are mainly due to anaphylaxis and so DOIC in anaphylaxis/anaphylactoid reactions is adrenaline. It is a type I or IgE mediated reactions.*

42. Thyroid uptake scan uses I^{123} and I^{131} $^{99m}T_c$ pertechnitate.
43. Regarding **mammographic** feature of C_A breast.

Benign Breast CA	*Malignant Breast CA.*
• Solid or lucent centered spherical lesion.	• Irregular speculated mass.
• Smooth and rounded calcifications.	• Clustered calcifications.
	• Smaller calcifications < 0.5 mm.
	• Architectural distortion.
• The size of calcification is > 1 mm in diameter.	• Focal asymmetric density.
• Structure/architecture well maintained.	

44. **Mammographically** MICROCALCIFICATION, focal areas of radiolucent densities and architectural distortion is characteristic of breast C_A.
45. Radiologic findings in **hydronephrosis** and **polycystic kidney** include dilatation of renal pelvis, uniformly enlarged renal shadow and distorted renal calyces.

> ***Note:*** *The main differentiating features in between them is **cysts** communicate with the pelvis in cases of hydronephrosis while in **PKD** it will not.*

46. The dose of radiotherapy recommended for pain relief in bone metastases is **30 Gy** in 10 fractions or **8 Gy** in one fraction.
47. A patient with cancer received extreme degree of radiation toxicity. Further history revealed that the dose adjustment of a particular drug was missed during the course of RT. The drug

required a dose adjustment in that patient during RT in order to prevent radiation toxicity is **Dactinomycin**.

48. The gold standard for the diagnosis of **osteoporosis** is **dual energy X-ray absorptiometry.**
49. **Angiographically**, the typical "beaded" or "pile of plates" appearance involving the internal carotid artery is observed as fibromuscular dysplasia.
50. After contrast media injection in the radiology department, a patient develops severe hypotension, bronchospasm and cyanosis. The drug should be used for treating this case is **Adrenaline**.
51. A patient is suspected to have **vestibular shwannoma**. The investigation of choice for its diagnosis is **gadolinium enhanced MRI**.
52. In **scurvy,** the **radiological signs** are seen include–
    - Pelican spur.
    - Zone of demarcation near epiphyses.
    - Fraenkel's line.
    - Trummer field zone.
    - Wimberger sign.
53. **Soap bubble appearance** is characteristically seen in **giant cell tumour** (osteoclastoma).
54. In **computed tomography (CT),** the attenuation values are measured in Hounsfield units (HU). An attenuation value of zero'0' HU corresponds to water (H_2O).

> ***Note:*** *HU for different medias are–*
> - *Air* – *minus (–) 1000 HU.*
> - *Water* – *zero (0) HU.*
> - *Dense bone* – *plus (+) 1000 HU.*

55. The **EEG cabins** should be completely shielded by a continuous sheet of wire mesh of copper to avoid the picking up of noise from external electromagnetic disturbances. Such a shielding is called as **FARADAY CAGE**.

56. The organs should always be imaged in a suspected case of bronchogenic C_A is **adrenal glands.**
57. A middle aged man presents with progressive atrophy and weakness of hand and forearms. On examination he is found to have slight spasticity of the leg, generalised hyper-reflexia and increased signal in the cortico-spinal tract on T_2-weighted MRI. The most likely diagnosis is **amyotrophic lateral sclerosis**.
58. A 6-year-old boy named Sultan has been complaining of headache, ignoring to see the objects on the side for four months. On examination, he is not mentally retarded, his grades at school are good, and visual acuity is diminished in both the eyes. Visual charting showed significant field defect. CT scan of the head showed suprasellar mass with calcification. The most probable diagnosis in this case is **CRANIOPHARYNGIOMA**.
59. A hepatic lesions that can be diagnosed with high accuracy by using nuclear imaging is **focal nodular hyperplasia (FNH)**.
60. The most beneficial technique of using chemotherapy with a course of radiotherapy in head and neck malignancies is **concomitant chemoradiotherapy**.
61. The techniques uses PIEZOELECTRIC CRYSTALS is **ultrasonography**.
62. The earliest radiographic manifestation of childhood leukaemia is **radioluscent transverse metaphyseal bands**.
63. Following are recognised examples of **Tumour markers**:
    - β-hCG.
    - α-fetoprotein.
    - Thyroglobulin.
    - β_2 microglobulin.
    - CEA.
    - PSA.
64. Cytogenetic abnormality associated with blood tumour:

Conditions	*Cytogenetic abnormality*
• AML–M3	(9:22)
• AML-myelodysplasia	(3:21)
• CML	t(9:22)
• Mantle cell lymphoma	(11:14)
• Follicular lymphoma	(14:18)
• Ewing's sarcoma	(22:21)
• Burkitt's lymphoma	(8:14)
• Papillary thyroid C_A	(10:17)

65. Early **gastric C_A** generally indicates that gastric adenocarcinoma confined to mucosa and submucosa.
66. **Migratory thrombophlebitis** is associated with lung C_A, pancreatic C_A and GIT C_A.

> ***Note:*** *It is rarely associated with prostatic C_A.*

67. Increased susceptibility of **breast CA** is likely to be associated with a mutation in **BRC_A-1 gene**.
68. A 7-year-old boy **Kalia** with left renal mass had bone pain and was detected to have bone metastatic deposits. The most likely renal tumour is → **clear cell sarcoma**.
69. **Badre Azam** a 55-year-old male presents with feature of obstructive jaundice. He also reports weight loss of 7 kg in last two months. On CAT scan, the CBD is dilated till the lower end and the main pancreatic duct is also dilated. Pancreas is normal. The most likely diagnosis is **Periampullary C_A**.
70. **Simmi**, a 20-year-old female patient presented with a thyroid swelling. Most probably the FNAC will not diagnose **follicular C_A of thyroid**.
71. **Ganami**, a 25-year-old male presents to emergency with history of road-traffic accident two hours ago. The patient is haemodynamically stable. Abdomen is soft. On catheterization of

the bladder, haematuria is noticed. The next step in the management should be contrast enhanced CAT scan of abdomen popularly called **CECT of abdomen**.

72. The investigation of choice for assessment of depth of penetration and perirectal nodes in rectal cancer is **Transrectal ultrasound**.

> ***Note:*** *Popularly called TRUS (Transrectal ultrasound) which is useful for staging of rectal cancer. It is almost free of radiation exposure risk.*

73. The most common pure malignant germ cell tumour of the ovary is **Dysgerminoma**.
74. The risk of complex hyperplasia of endometrium with atypia progressing to malignancy in a postmenopausal woman is **28%**.
75. The treatment of choice in renal cell C_A with the tumour of less than 4 cm in size is **partial nephrectomy**.
76. **Ramkali Bai**, a 36-year-old female presented with one year history of menstrual irregularity and galactorrhoea. She also had off and on headache. Her examination revealed bitemporal superior quadrantopia. Her fundus examination showed primary optic atrophy. The most likely diagnosis here is **pituitary macroadenoma**.
77. Regarding **kidney transplantation**–
    - Renal transplantation is autotrophic.
    - Cyclosporine is the mainstay of immunosuppression others used like antithymocyte globulin, Tacrolinus and azathioprine.
    - Kidney after removal is flushed with cold perfusion solution.
    - There are 2 types of kidney preservation (i) Cold storage and (ii) Machine perfusion.
78. **Bhagat Pandey**, a 42-year-old patient is suffering from carotid body tumour. The best choice for treatment here is **excision of tumour**.
79. Recognised indication of postoperative RT in a case of C_A endometrium includes:

- Myometrial invasion > ½ thickness.
- Positive lymph nodes.
- Endocervical involvement.

80. **5 HT** is increased in **Carcinoid syndrome**.
81. In a clear cell C_A of kidney with a solitary pulmonary metastasis, proceed with removal of diseased kidney.
82. **Brodie's grading of tumours** pertains to histological differentiation.
83. Cancer cells derive their energy primarily from → **Anaerobic glycolysis**.
84. **Farida**, a 33-year-old patient is diagnosed with C_A breast. The most important prognostic factor in the treatment of this disease is → **Axillary metastases**.
85. **Transvaginal US** with Doppler colour flow imaging is used to detect malignant ovarian tumours on the basis of the neovascularity of tumour blood supply.

> **Note:** *It is used, infact, to detect ovarian tumour at an early stage.*

86. While bathing her 2-year-old son named **Golu**, a mother feel a mass in his abdomen. A thorough medical evaluation of the child reveals aniridia, hypospadius, horseshoe kidney, and hemihypetrophy. The most likely diagnosis is **Wilms' tumour**.
87. In **Dysgerminomas**, the propensity for lymphatic invasion is great.
88. The **median age of patient** with **endodermal sinus tumour** or **Yolk sac tumour** is **19 years**. The classic histologic findings is the **Schiller-Duval body**, a central vessel lined with columnar cells.
89. **Tamoxifen** acts as an antioestrogen in the breast but stimulates the endometrium similarly to oestrogen, resulting in an increased risk of endometrial C_A (relative risk of 7).

90. In C_AC_X **cases,** colposcopically directed biopsies carry an accuracy of **85 to 95%.**
91. The **median age** for **endometrial** C_A is **61 years**. The greatest number of patient is between **50 and 59 years of age.**
92. **TET Scan** technique is the best for differentiating recurrence of brain tumour from radiation therapy induced necrosis.
93. The most radiosensitive tumour is **Ewings tumour/sarcoma.**
94. Investigation of choice for detection and characterization of interstitial lung disease is **High resolution CT scan.**
95. The most common cause of sclerotic skeletal metastasis in a female patient is **Breast** C_A.
96. The most common cause of a mixed cystical solid suprasellar mass seen on cranial MRI scan of a 10-year-old child is **CRANIOPHARYNGIOMA.**
97. The most common inherited malignancy is **Retinoblastoma**.
98. **Gastrin** is a biochemical marker for pancreatic neuroendocrine tumour (Gastrinoma or Zollinger-Ellison syndrome).
99. The most common pituitary adenoma is **Prolactinoma.**
100. Lung to lung metastases is seen in **Adenocarcinoma lung.**
101. **Cerebral cortical degeneration** is not a non-metastatic complication of malignancies.
102. The most common site of metastatic disease is **lung.**
103. **Hypercalcemia** associated with malignancy is most often mediated by parathyroid hormone related protein (PTHr P).
104. **Tumour lysis syndrome** has hypocalcemia not hypercalcemia.
105. The most common paraneoplastic syndrome is → **Hypercalcemia.**

106. The clinical conditions commonly predisposes to colonic C_A is → **Ulcerative colitis.**
107. Pancreatitis, pituitary tumour and phacochromocytoma may be associated with → **Medullary C_A of thyroid.**
108. **Gardner's syndrome** is a rare AD hereditary disorder involving colon and is characterized by polyposis in jejunum, pituitary adenoma and skin tumours.
109. The overall survival is increased by screening procedure in **colonic C_A.**
110. **Carcinoid tumour** with highest incidence of metastases is from **Pancreatic carcinoid**.
111. Incidence of carcinoid syndrome is maximum with Appendix carcinoid:

Note: *The 2nd common is pancreas.*

112. Recognised **testicular tumour marker** includes—AFP, LCG, and LDH. Besides PLAP and GGTP is also included here.
113. A soft tissue sarcomas frequently metastasizes to lymph nodes is → **Embryonal rhabdomyosarcoma.**
114. **Gastrin** is a biochemical marker for pancreatic neuroendocrine tumour (Gastrinoma or Zollinger-Ellison syndrome).
115. The tissue of origin of the Kaposi's sarcoma is **Vascular.**